T0364793

Rotator Cuff Deficiency of the Shoulder

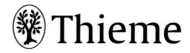

Rotator Cuff Deficiency of the Shoulder

Mark A. Frankle, MD
Chief
Shoulder and Elbow Sugery
Florida Orthopaedic Institute Research Foundation
Temple Terrace, Florida

Thieme
New York • Stuttgart

Thieme Medical Publishers, Inc.
333 Seventh Ave.
New York, NY 10001

Editor: Esther Gumpert
Managing Editor: Owen Zurhellen IV
Vice President, Production and Electronic Publishing: Anne T. Vinnicombe
Production Editor: Print Matters
Vice President International Marketing and Sales: Cornelia Schulze
Chief Financial Officer: Peter van Woerden
President: Brian D. Scanlan
Medical Illustrator: Peggy Firth
Compositor: Compset, Inc.
Printer: Everbest Printing Company, Ltd

Library of Congress Cataloging-in-Publication Data

Rotator cuff deficiency of the shoulder / [edited by] Mark A. Frankle.
        p. ; cm.
    Includes bibliographical references and index.
    ISBN 978-1-58890-506-2 (tpn : alk. paper)
        1.   Shoulder joint—Rotator cuff—Diseases.   I.   Frankle, Mark A.
    [DNLM: 1. Rotator Cuff—surgery. 2. Arthroscopy. 3. Joint Prosthesis. 4. Rotator Cuff—injuries. WE 810 R8417 2008]
    RD557.5.R669 2008
    617.4'720597—dc22

                                                                                                    2007044534

Important note: Medical knowledge is ever-changing. As new research and clinical experience broaden our knowledge, changes in treatment and drug therapy may be required. The authors and editors of the material herein have consulted sources believed to be reliable in their efforts to provide information that is complete and in accord with the standards accepted at the time of publication. However, in view of the possibility of human error by the authors, editors, or publisher of the work herein or changes in medical knowledge, neither the authors, editors, or publisher, nor any other party who has been involved in the preparation of this work, warrants that the information contained herein is in every respect accurate or complete, and they are not responsible for any errors or omissions or for the results obtained from use of such information. Readers are encouraged to confirm the information contained herein with other sources. For example, readers are advised to check the product information sheet included in the package of each drug they plan to administer to be certain that the information contained in this publication is accurate and that changes have not been made in the recommended dose or in the contraindications for administration. This recommendation is of particular importance in connection with new or infrequently used drugs.

Some of the product names, patents, and registered designs referred to in this book are in fact registered trademarks or proprietary names even though specific reference to this fact is not always made in the text. Therefore, the appearance of a name without designation as proprietary is not to be construed as a representation by the publisher that it is in the public domain.

Printed in China

5 4 3 2 1

ISBN   978-1-58890-506-2

Contents

Foreword

Rotator cuff problems are the most common source of shoulder pain, and as such are thoughtfully included in the diagnostic evaluation of patients presenting with shoulder pain. A tremendous spectrum of injury and disease affects the rotator cuff. The list of issues is almost too long to enumerate, including strain, inflammation, abrasion, partial tearing with tear sizes extending from small to extra-large, and acute or chronic full-thickness tearing. Related issues involving the long-headed biceps, degenerative changes on the acromion process or hypertrophic enlargement of the acromioclavicular joint, stiffness or instability, and varying degrees of associated arthritic involvement of the glenohumeral joint also affect the rotator cuff. One can spend an entire professional career studying these various areas and trying to reach conclusions about the best treatment utilizing current knowledge.

Over the last several decades, a revolution has occurred. The introduction of arthroscopy and the development of arthroscopic surgical tools have created an entirely new approach to dealing with rotator cuff problems. Magnetic resonance imaging has allowed visualization of details of the rotator cuff and its musculature that was heretofore not possible. A new type of shoulder prosthesis has been introduced to replace not only arthritic joint surfaces but also a deficient rotator cuff. Earlier attempts at this had been inconsistent with limited effectiveness. However, now there is promise that a new implant, the reverse type of shoulder prosthesis, will have the necessary consistency and effectiveness to become a first-line treatment choice for patients with concordant rotator cuff deficiency, substantial arthritis, and usually a lack of active motion away from the side.

Dr. Mark A. Frankle, the editor of this book, is an extremely energetic champion to further the understanding of the rotator cuff deficient shoulder and its treatment. He has brought together a magnificent set of chapters by authors with unparalleled scientific background and practical experience. For example, Professor Kai-Nan An has authored hundreds of peer-reviewed manuscripts on the biomechanics of the upper extremity, and he codifies his understanding of these concepts in the introductory chapter. Other scholarly authors bring to the book focused information on epidemiology and natural history, conservative treatment, arthroscopic initiatives, muscle replacement, tendon replacement, and the thoughtful reminder of the full spectrum of disease that can occur within this area. The main subject, cuff tear arthropathy, is introduced with a thorough discussion of classification systems defining the various components of this problem. In considering prosthetic replacement, the tried-and-true role of hemiarthroplasty is presented with its great benefits and its striking limitations as well. The coup de grâce, though, is the magnificently expansive discussion of the rational and mechanics for the reverse shoulder prosthesis. This is coupled with exposition of the clinical experience from four centers. These unaltered opinions side by side allow the reader to compare and contrast viewpoints—something that just cannot be done in scientific journals, but only in a textbook setting.

We are all well schooled in the concepts of evolution and the supposition that things slowly change over time. In fact, the changes are uneven in magnitude and have no set schedule. The quite dramatic, rapid changes that have occurred in this area may have been completed in our professional lifetimes. As we are unable to predict the future with any degree of accuracy, I think we all must believe that the material included in this text may endure for quite some time. Congratulations to Dr. Frankle for developing the concept for this book so wonderfully and to all the authors for helping us to better understand rotator cuff deficiencies and their myriad manifestations of presentation and nuances for treatment.

Robert H. Cofield, MD
Caywood Professor of Orthopaedics
Mayo Clinic College of Medicine
Consultant in Orthopaedic Surgery
Mayo Clinic
Rochester, Minnesota

Preface

In the early 21st century, the diseases faced by developed nations have begun to shift. The number of people who are over 50 years of age will soon outnumber those under 50. This demographic change will correspondingly increase the disease burden in this segment of the aging population. It is estimated that once a person reaches the age of 65, he or she has a 50% chance of developing a torn rotator cuff. The millions of people already affected by rotator cuff disease has accounted for billions of dollars in health-care costs to diagnose and treat this problem. Additionally, the economic impact of disabled workers due to rotator cuff injuries cannot be overstated. Although the majority of these patients are able to be treated conventionally for repairable rotator cuff tears, there exists an ever-increasing number of patients faced with an irreparable tear. Many of these people are often given confusing information regarding their options and are offered treatments unlikely to help. As a result, they may increase their pain and diminish their shoulder function.

This situation has evolved from a combination of factors including our inability as physicians to recognize when these tears are beyond repair with conventional methods and our reluctance to recognize the increasing magnitude of the problem, which suggests a course of benign neglect. To stop this problem, we must identify nonoperative treatments that compensate for the rotator cuff defect and consider operative treatments such as reconstructive surgery. To this end, I have recruited physicians from around the world who have demonstrated their authority on the successful treatment of patients with a rotator cuff–deficient shoulder. The historical perspective, classification, and nonoperative and operative management of rotator cuff disease of various well-known institutions is shared within several unique chapters. It is my hope that this book will be helpful to orthopedic surgeons who focus on treating patients with shoulder problems by providing an array of successful treatment methodologies.

Acknowledgment

For their efforts, I would like to acknowledge all the contributing authors and the research group at the Florida Orthopaedic Institute Research Foundation led by Derek Pupello, whose help has been immeasurable.

partial-thickness tear increased intratendinous strain for all joint abduction positions except 15 degrees.[21]

The strains on the joint and bursal sides of the supraspinatus tendon with increasing load and during glenohumeral abduction were quantified using extensometers.[22] Increasing the tendon load increased the strains on the joint side significantly more than on the bursal side. During glenohumeral abduction, the strain of tissue on the joint side increased progressively, but on the bursal side, it decreased beyond 60 degrees of elevation. It was speculated that the differential strain may cause shearing between the layers of the supraspinatus tendon, and thus be a causative factor in failure of the supraspinatus tendon. Using the same experimental technique, the potential propagation of thickness tears was also examined. With a simulated full-thickness tear of the tendon midsubstance, the strain on the bursal side increased with load and elevation angles. An intratendinous delamination tear increased joint-side strain during abduction and bursal-side strain with loading. Tear propagation was observed from joint to bursal sides during abduction. Eventually, the tendon failure occurred at the insertion.[23]

The strain in the model within the repaired RC tendon decreased significantly with the arm elevated more than 30 degrees. The strain increased in IR and decreased in ER. It was concluded that more than 30 degrees of elevation in the coronal or scapular plane and rotation ranging from 0 degrees to 60 degrees of ER compose the safe range of motion (ROM) after repair of the RC.[24]

The Rotator Cuff as Joint Stabilizer

Even though the glenohumeral joint has a large ROM, it is still stable. The joint consists of the intercalated joint surfaces of the humeral head and glenoid, along with the surrounding capsuloligamentous structures. Interaction between the capsuloligamentous structures and the articulating surfaces provides the basic static constraint of the joint. On the contrary, coordinated muscle contraction provides the dynamic balance and stability of the joint.

The concavity of the glenoid surface provides constraint to the joint under compressive force.[25] Compression into the glenoid labral concavity keeps the humeral head centered. The constraining mechanism of concavity-compression was quantified by translating the glenoid underneath the humeral head in eight different directions.[26] Relative translations between the glenoid and the humeral head and the forces resisting translation were recorded. The stability ratio, defined as the peak translational force divided by the applied compressive force, was calculated. The results indicated that stability ratios were 56, 60, 32, and 37% in the superior, inferior, anterior, and posterior directions, respectively. Removal of the glenoid labrum resulted in an average decrease in stability ratio of 9.6%. Even moderate compressive forces generated by the RC are sufficient to provide stability through the concavity-compression mechanism.

Muscle acts three-dimensionally to the distal bony segment across the joint. All muscle force vectors can be resolved into compressive and shear components (**Fig. 1–3**). For the RC muscle at the glenohumeral joint, the dominant component of force was perpendicular to the glenoid surface. This compressive force generated by each of the RC muscles changed significantly with the axial humeral rotation. In neutral rotation, the compressive force component averaged 90, 85, 98, and 96% of the muscle force in the teres minor, infraspinatus, subscapularis, and supraspinatus, respectively. The compressive component of the muscle force stabilizes the glenohumeral joint through the mechanism of concavity-compression as described earlier.

The shear component of the muscle force could either stabilize or destabilize the joint by direct pull. The direction and magnitude of the shear force in anterior, posterior, superior, and inferior directions generated by each RC muscle were relatively small compared with the compressive component. They also changed significantly with humeral rotation. Anterior shear force components by the

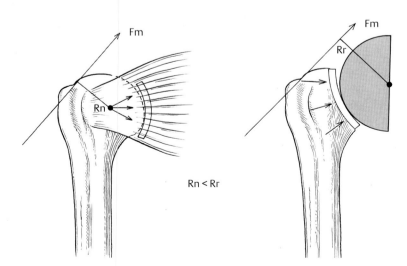

Figure 1–3 Superior view of the shoulder. Muscle acts three-dimensionally to the distal bony segment across the joint. All muscle force vectors can be resolved into compressive and shear components. The compressive component of the muscle force stabilizes the glenohumeral joint through the mechanism of concavity-compression. The shear component of the muscle force could either stabilize or destabilize the joint by direct pull.

teres minor (19%) and infraspinatus (16%) in neutral rotation changed to posterior shear forces (5 and 8%) in 90 degrees ER. The supraspinatus generated destabilizing anterior shear force as high as 31% of the applied force to the muscle in 90 degrees ER, which was significantly different from the other muscles in this position.

To facilitate the comparison of stabilizing/destabilizing roles of RC muscles, the dynamic stability index was considered. This index was defined by considering both the effects due to concavity-compression mechanism as well as the shear force generated by the muscle. It represented the percentage of the unit muscle force in constraining the joint subluxation.[27] The dynamic stability index in the anterior direction, for example, was significantly different when the humerus was in neutral rotation (13, 13 47, and 60% for teres minor, infraspinatus, supraspinatus, and subscapularis, respectively) compared with the end-ROM at 90 degrees of ER (37, 41, 0, and 32% for teres minor, infraspinatus, supraspinatus, and subscapularis, respectively).

Principles of Reversed Total Shoulder Arthroplasty for Severe Rotator Cuff Tear Arthropathy

The application of reversed total shoulder arthroplasty is becoming popular in treating patients with severe cuff tear arthropathy. The basic concept involved in such design is related to the shift of the center of joint rotation so that the lever arms of the remaining muscle, such as the deltoid, could be more effectively functional. In general, the center of joint rotation is located at the center of curvature of the articular surface in spinning motion (**Fig. 1–4**). In the normal shoulder, the center of rotation is located in the center of convex surface of the humeral head. In the reversed total shoulder, the convex surface is placed on the glenoid side. The center of curvature, and thus the center of rotation, is located in the glenoid component, which is further away from the deltoid muscle. Therefore, an increased lever arm for more effective function of the muscle is expected.

The application of reversed total shoulder arthroplasty has another advantage in terms of implant fixation. The implant fixation for the glenoid component is usually more critical and difficult compared with that in the humeral head due to the inferior bony stock. In general, assuming that the joint articular surface is frictionless, the joint contact forces are perpendicular to the joint surface (**Fig. 1–4**) and are directed to the center of curvature. In the normal shoulder joint or arthroplasty, the joint contact force would

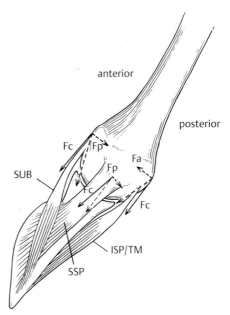

Figure 1–4 The application of reversed total shoulder arthroplasty, in treating severe cuff tear arthropathy, would shift the center of joint rotation so that the lever arms of the remaining muscle could be more effectively functional. In addition, the joint contact forces are perpendicular to the joint surface and are directed to the center of curvature. In the normal shoulder joint or arthroplasty, the joint contact force would apply to the glenoid surface in an eccentric manner. In that condition, the so-called rocking horse effect may be experienced. However, in the reversed total shoulder arthroplasty, the contact force on the glenoid component is more in the concentric manner pointing to the center of curvature where the peg of fixation is located to resist the loading.

apply to the glenoid surface in an eccentric manner. In that condition, the so-called rocking horse effect may be experienced and could lead to implant loosening. However, in the reversed total shoulder arthroplasty, the contact force on the glenoid component is more in the concentric manner pointing to the center of curvature where the peg of fixation is located to resist the loading. Therefore, the loading in the glenoid component would be more favorable in this reversed total shoulder replacement.

Conclusion

The rotator cuff muscles play an important role in moving and stabilizing the glenohumeral joint. The line of action and movement of the muscles are important biomechanical factors that need to be considered in the treatment of associated pathologies of rotator cuff tear.

References

1. Bassett R, Browne A, Morrey B, An K. Glenohumeral muscle force and moment mechanics in a position of shoulder instability. J Biomech 1990;23(5):405–415

2. Keating J, Waterworth P, Shaw-Dunn J, Corssan J. The relative strengths of the rotator cuff muscles. A cadaver study. J Bone Joint Surg Br 1993;75-B:137–140

3. An K, Ueba Y, Chao E, Cooney W, Linscheid R. Tendon excursion and moment arm of index finger muscles. J Biomech 1983;16:419–425

4. Otis J, Jiang C, Wickiewicz T, Peterson M, Warren R, Santner TJ. Changes in the moment arms of the rotator cuff and deltoid muscles with abduction and rotation. J Bone Joint Surg Am 1994;76(5):667–676

5. Kuechle D, Newman S, Itoi E, Morrey B, An K. Shoulder muscle moment arms during horizontal flexion and elevation. J Shoulder Elbow Surg 1997;6(5):429–439

6. Kuechle D, Newman S, Itoi E, Niebur G, Morrey B, An K. The relevance of the moment arm of shoulder muscles with respect to axial rotation of the glenohumeral joint in four positions. Clin Biomech (Bristol, Avon) 2000;15(5):322–329

7. Halder A, O'Driscoll S, Heers G, et al. Biomechanical comparison of effects of supraspinatus tendon detachments, tendon defects, and muscle retractions. J Bone Joint Surg Am 2002;84-A(5):780–785

8. Mura N, O'Driscoll S, Zobitz M, et al. The effect of infraspinatus disruption on glenohumeral torque and superior migration of the humeral head: a biomechanical study. J Shoulder Elbow Surg 2003;12(2):179–184

9. Liu J, Hughes R, O'Driscoll S, An K. Biomechanical effect of medial advancement of the supraspinatus tendon. J Bone Joint Surg Am 1998;80A(6):853–860

10. Nakajima T, Lee S, Hughes R, O'Driscoll S, An K. Abduction moment arm of transposed subscapularis tendon. Clin Biomech (Bristol, Avon) 1999;14(4):265–270

11. Mura N, O'Driscoll S, Zobitz M, Heers G, An K. Biomechanical effect of a patch graft for large rotator cuff tears: a cadaver study. Clin Orthop Relat Res 2003;415:131–138

12. Itoi E, Berglund L, Grabowski J, et al. Tensile properties of the supraspinatus tendon. J Orthop Res 1995;13(4):578–584

13. Nakajima T, Rokuuma N, Hamada K, Tomatsu T, Fukuda H. Histologic and biomechanical characteristics of the supraspinatus tendon: Reference to rotator cuff tearing. J Shoulder Elbow Surg 1994;3:79–87

14. Halder A, Zobitz M, Schultz F, An K. Mechanical properties of the posterior rotator cuff. Clin Biomech (Bristol, Avon) 2000;15:456–462

15. Halder A, Zobitz M, Schultz F, An K. Structural properties of the subscapularis tendon. J Orthop Res 2000;18(5):829–834

16. Lee S, Nakajima T, Luo Z, Zobitz M , Chang Y, An K . The bursal and articular sides of the supraspinatus tendon have a different compressive stiffness. Clin Biomech (Bristol, Avon) 2000;15(4):241–247

17. Nightingale E, Allen C, Sonnabend D, Goldberg J, Walksh W. Mechanical properties of the rotator cuff: response to cyclic loading at varying abduction angles. Knee Surg Sports Traumatol Arthrosc 2003;11(6):389–392

18. Luo Z, Hsu H, Grabowski J, Morrey B, An K. Mechanical environment associated with rotator cuff tears. J Shoulder Elbow Surg 1998;7(5):616–620

19. Wakabayashi I, Itoi E, Sano H, et al. Mechanical environment of the supraspinatus tendon: a two-dimensional finite element model analysis. J Shoulder Elbow Surg 2003;12(6):612–617

20. Bey M, Song HK, Wehrli F, Soslowsky L. Intratendinous strain fields of the intact supraspinatus tendon: The effect of glenohumeral joint position and tendon region. J Orthop Res 2002;20(4):869–874

21. Bey M, Ramsey M, Soslowsky L. Intratendinous strain fields of the supraspinatus tendon: effect of a surgically created articular-surface rotator cuff tear. J Shoulder Elbow Surg 2002;11(6):562–569

22. Reilly P, Amis A, Wallace A, Emery R. Mechanical factors in the initiation and propagation of tears of the rotator cuff. Quantification of strains of the supraspinatus tendon in vitro. J Bone Joint Surg Br 2003;85-B(4):594–599

23. Reilly P, Amis A, Wallace A, Emery R. Supraspinatus tears: propagation and strain alteration. J Shoulder Elbow Surg 2003;12(2):134–138

24. Hatakeyama Y, Itoi E, Pradhan R, Urayama M, Sato K. Effect of arm elevation and rotation on the strain in the repaired rotator cuff tendon. A cadaveric study. Am J Sports Med 2001;29(6):788–794

25. Lazarus M, Sidles J, Harryman D, Matsen F. Effect of a chondrallabral defect on glenoid concavity and glenohumeral stability. A cadaveric model. J Bone Joint Surg Am 1996;78:94–102.

26. Halder A, Kuhl S, Zobitz M, Larson D, An K. Effects of the glenoid labrum and glenohumeral abduction on stability of the shoulder joint through concavity-compression: an in vitro study. J Bone Joint Surg Am 2001;83:1062–1069

27. Lee S, Kim K, O'Driscoll S, Morrey B, An K. Dynamic glenohumeral stability provided by the rotator cuff muscles in the mid-range and end-range of motion. J Bone Joint Surg Am 2000;82:849–857

2 Massive Irreparable Rotator Cuff Tears

Mark Mighell

The etiology of massive rotator cuff tears is multifactorial and continues to be a researched topic. To understand this topic requires a basic knowledge of rotator cuff (RC) histopathology.

Anatomy of the Rotator Cuff

A clear understanding of the normal anatomy of the RC will aid in the treatment of the diseased cuff. Clark and Harryman[1] have described the RC in detail. From their work, we know that as the tendons of the posterior cuff approach their site of insertion, they are confluent and not easily separated. Their studies have shown that the RC is made up of multiple, confluent tissue layers functioning in concert.

Histological sections through the supraspinatus and infraspinatus reveal five distinct layers (**Fig. 2–1**). The most superficial layer contains large arterioles and comprises fibers from the coracohumeral ligament. A sheet of fibrous tissue from the coracohumeral ligament's origin extends posterolaterally to form a sheet over the supraspinatus and infraspinatus. This layer is 1 mm in thickness and the tissue fibers are oriented obliquely to the long axis of the muscle bellies. Layer 2 is 3- to 5-mm thick and represents the direct tendinous insertion into the tuberosities. Large bundles of densely packed parallel tendon fibers compose this layer. Layer 3 is ~3-mm thick and comprises smaller bundles of collagen with a less uniform organization. Fibers within this layer travel at 45-degree angles to one another to form an interdigitating meshwork that contributes to the fusion of the cuff tendon insertion. Layer 4 comprises loose connective tissue and thick collagen bands that merge with the coracohumeral ligament at the most anterior border of the supraspinatus. Layer 5 (2-mm thick) represents the shoulder capsule. With respect to the blood supply, the arterioles are larger and the vessels more prevalent on the bursal surface of the cuff and branch between layers 2 and 3.[1] The articular side of the RC is relatively hypovascular when compared with the rich blood flow on the bursal side of the cuff.[2]

Histologically, tendon regions subject almost exclusively to tension differ from those exposed to high levels of compression as well as tension.[3] Tendons not subject to compression consist primarily of spindle-shaped fibroblasts surrounded by densely packed, longitudinally oriented collagen fibers principally made up of type I collagen. In contrast, tendons exposed to compression have a fibrocartilaginous structure and a composition characterized by rounded cells surrounded by a matrix contain-

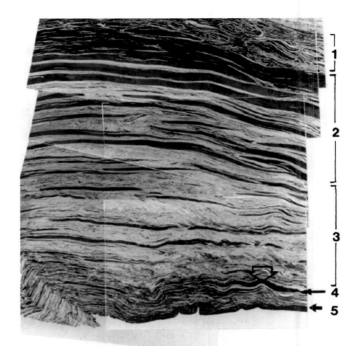

Figure 2–1 Vertical, transverse section through the supraspinatus tendon and capsule near the tendon insertion. Layer 1 is composed of fibers of the coracohumeral ligament obliquely oriented with respect to the axis of each muscle. Large arterioles are present. Layer 2 is composed of closely packed parallel tendon fibers grouped in large bundles. Layer 3 has smaller fascicles and these fascicles lack a uniform orientation. Blood vessels are also present in this layer, but are smaller than those in layers 1 and 2. Layer 4 is composed of loose connective tissue in which there are thick bands of collagen fibers. The only blood vessels in this layer are capillaries, found adjacent to the extraarticular surface of the capsule of the shoulder. Layer 5 is a thin, continuous sheet of interwoven collagen fibrils, which usually insert on the humerus as Sharpey's fibers within the bone.

ing type I and type II collagen, chondroitan-4-sulfate, and chondroitan-6-sulfate.[4]

Prevalence

Degeneration of the RC is a common source of shoulder dysfunction. It has been demonstrated that the presence of RC pathology was highly predictive of impaired physical health and quality of life.[5-7] In fact, the size of this impact is comparable to the effects of conditions such as diabetes mellitus, myocardial infarction, congestive heart failure, hypertension, and clinical depression.[6]

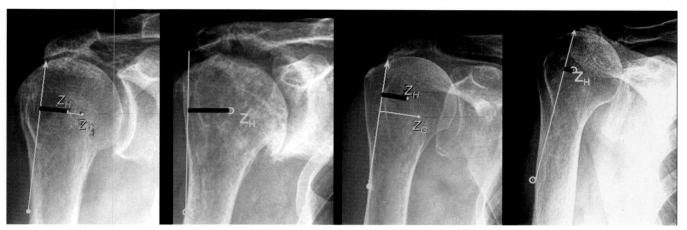

Figure 3–3 Typical x-rays of the four types of rotator cuff tear arthropathy according to the author's classification (*Bar:* lever of the deltoid)

balance of the force couple of the subscapularis in the front and the infraspinatus in the back as counterpart of the superior displacing effect of the strong deltoid muscle (**Fig. 3–2**).

Author's Classification System

The specific problems and features of single etiologies are extensively described in the previous chapter. Besides the specific problems, there is a common feature for all pathologies that is characterized by a progressive soft tissue and bone defect, which causes superior migration and instability of the humeral head. Because of this, we developed a more biomechanical, functional, and morphologic classification, which focuses on the position and stability of the center of rotation of the glenohumeral joint (**Fig. 3–3**).[21,22]

In developing our classification as a tool in decision making for prosthetic therapy of CTA, our criteria were as follows:

–Not a simple pathomorphologic description

–Biomechanically oriented

–Description amount of static and dynamic anterosuperior instability

–Position and stability of center of rotation as decisive parameters

–Therapeutically oriented

–Independent from underlying pathology

–Additional tool for decision making in prosthetic treatment *beside* the clinical parameters

Therefore, we established a mainly functional and biomechanical classification of CTAs into four types focusing on the position and stability of the center of rotation on static (normal x-ray) and dynamic (fluoroscopy) radiologic investigations. In types Ia and Ib, the center of rotation is not displaced, whereas in types IIa and IIb it is significantly cranially displaced. Type IIb is characterized by a complete static or dynamic anterosuperior instability (**Table 3–1**).

Sometimes it is difficult to distinguish between types IIa and IIb on a simple static anteroposterior x-ray. To distinguish between both types the clinical aspect under loaded conditions (active abduction or elevation against resistance) shows an increased superior displacement in type IIb patients. This could be also proved by a radiologic investigation under fluoroscopy (**Fig. 3–4**).

The four types are markedly different in respect to preoperative function after elimination of pain and to the results after conventional shoulder hemiarthroplasty.[23]

Treatment of Rotator Cuff Tear Arthropathy by Shoulder Arthroplasty

Current Options

Different approaches to the treatment of defect arthropathies (osteoarthritis with irreparable cuff defects) are de-

Table 3–1 Pathomechanics and Pathomorphologic Classification of Cuff Tear Arthropathy

Type Ia	Type Ib	Type IIa	Type IIb
Centered, stable	Centered, medialized	Decentered, limited stability	Decentered, unstable
No superior migration	No superior migration	Superior translation	Anterosuperior dislocation
Acetabularization of coracoacromial arch; femoralization of humeral head	Medial erosion of the glenoid	Minimum stabilization by coracoacromial arch	No stabilization by coracoacromial arch

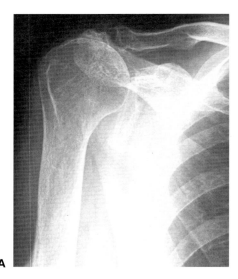

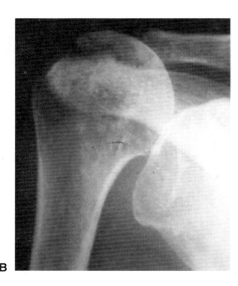

Figure 3–4 Anteroposterior x-ray, static and dynamic with fluoroscopy: **(A)** superior displacement with the arm resting at the side, and **(B)** superior dislocation with the arm under resisted abduction.

scribed in the literature. The use of conventional anatomical prostheses leads at best to an alleviation of pain. Functional results to be expected have already been described by Neer as "limited goal rehabilitation."[24] The often contradictory results of hemiarthroplasty have been analyzed prospectively by Wirth et al.[25] Poor functional results can be expected if the cuff is not reconstructed, is irreparable, or if the restraint of the coracoacromial arch is lacking. Even with the use of big or oversized humeral heads in special cases, the results are at best satisfactory.[26,27] Constraint prostheses introduced at the end of the 1970s and the beginning of the 1980s have been abandoned because of early loosening.[28] In addition, the functional results of the bipolar prostheses are definitively less uniform and reach, at best, the outcome of the reversed prosthesis in their lower quarter results (in general, multiply-operated patients with often-damaged deltoid muscles).[29,30] With the exception of the constraint prosthesis, the reason for these poor results of hemiarthroplasties and bipolar prostheses is that the center of rotation is not brought sufficiently caudal and medial. This is necessary to optimize the function of the deltoid.

Even if the normal center of rotation has been restored, the functional results are not as good as those with the reverse prosthesis (**Fig. 3--5**). For this reason, the aforementioned prosthesis can be used for type I defect arthropathies accompanied by significant medial glenoid erosion (type Ib of our classification). The use of oversized humeral heads during hemiarthroplasty leads more to a lateralization than to a lowering of the center of rotation and that deteriorates the moment of rotation of the deltoid muscle. Reports dealing with hemiarthroplasties or bipolar prostheses list their results as excellent and good, even when the maximal elevation and abduction do not exceed 110 degrees.[25–31]

Outcome Depending on Our Classification

To evaluate the practicability and usefulness of our classification, we did a retrospective analysis on 37 (10 men, 27 women) patients with large and massive cuff tears (minimally involved two tendons) and concomitant degenera-

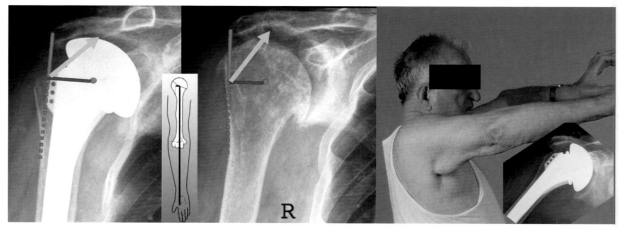

Figure 3–5 Acceptable clinical result with an anatomic hemiarthroplasty for a type Ib defect.

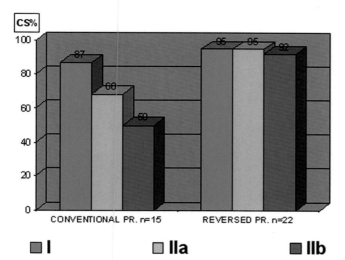

Figure 3–6 Retrospective study of result of rotator cuff tear arthropathy treated with hemiarthroplasty versus reversed shoulder arthroplasty in correlation to the types of rotator cuff tear arthropathy according to author's classification. Clinical results are shown as median of an age- and sex-corrected Constant Score.[32]

correlation of the Constant Score in the hemiarthroplasty group with the type of cuff-tear arthropathy graded to our classification system. In the patient group treated with the reverse shoulder arthroplasty, no outcome difference could be found between the different types of CTA (**Fig. 3–6**). In the type IIa and IIb groups, we treated 5 of the 15 hemiarthroplasty patients with an extra-large modular head. This subgroup did not have a better clinical outcome. The estimated biomechanical advantage of the large heads was not seen and clinically, the results tended to be worse than with anatomically sized heads due to overstuffing of the soft tissue envelope (**Fig. 3–7**).

To prove our results, we did a prospective study on 63 patients with massive and irreparable RC tear and degenerative or inflammatory changes of the glenohumeral joint. Due to the bad results in the retrospective study, type IIb patients only were treated with reversed shoulder arthroplasty (**Fig. 3–8**). Because of the poor glenoid bone stock type, type Ib patients never were treated with reversed shoulder prosthesis (**Fig. 3–5**). The patients were operated on between January 2000 and June 2002. Twelve patients received a modular conventional hemiarthroplasty (Global Shoulder System) with a "size-adapted" 5-head or a CTA 7-head. Six patients were treated with bipolar prostheses and 46 patients were treated with reversed prostheses Delta III. The average age of 70 years and the sex distribution (male: female = 1:3) were both the same as in the retrospective study. After a mean follow-up of 14 months, the Constant Score (age and sex corrected) was recorded. The results (**Table 3–2**) were very similar to the retrospective study.

Similar to the retrospective study, significantly worse results with conventional arthroplasty than with reversed arthroplasty in the type IIa could be found. This is clearly

tive or inflammatory joint disease. Patients were operated between 1993 and 1999. Fifteen patients were treated with a modular hemiarthroplasty (Global Shoulder System, DePuy Inc., Warsaw, IN), 5 of the 15 patients got an oversized extra-large head. Twenty-two patients did receive a reverse shoulder arthroplasty (Delta III, Global Shoulder System, DePuy Inc., Warsaw, IN). The mean age of the patients was 70 years. The clinical result after a minimum of 2-year follow-up was documented in an age- and sex-corrected Constant Score[32] (CS%). There was a significant

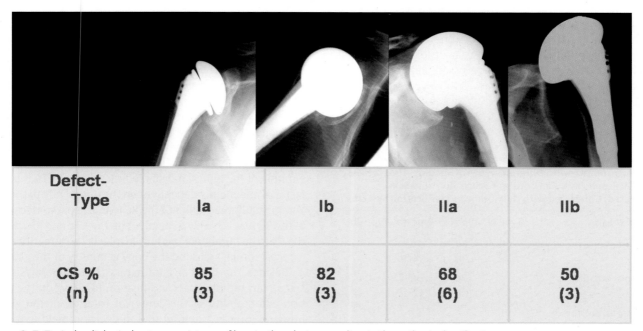

Defect-Type	Ia	Ib	IIa	IIb
CS % (n)	85 (3)	82 (3)	68 (6)	50 (3)

Figure 3–7 Typical radiological outcome pictures of hemiarthroplasty according to the author's classification.

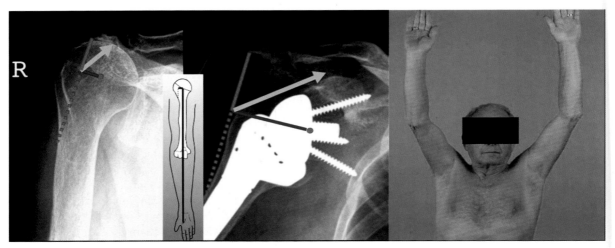

Figure 3–8 Excellent clinical result with a reversed arthroplasty for a type IIb defect.

related to the unfavorable biomechanical circumstances in these patients. The fact of a high and unstable position of the center of rotation weakens the deltoid as the mainly functioning muscle around the joint. The best results were found in the type IIb group treated with reversed arthroplasty (**Fig. 3–8**).

Conclusions

Despite favorable clinical short- and midterm clinical results[33,34] with the current reverse shoulder prostheses, recent studies have reported an increased percentage of inferior glenoid erosion and higher rates of revision after 6 to 7 years of follow-up.[35] Hence, the use of a reversed shoulder arthroplasty for all patients with a pathological glenohumeral joint and a concomitant large or massive RC tear cannot be recommended. The age of the patients is the most decisive parameter for differential indication in arthroplasty for CTA. Until 10-year or longer follow-up studies are known, the use of reversed shoulder arthroplasties in patients younger than 70 to 75 years old should be discussed seriously.

Table 3–2   Prospective Comparative Study of Treatment of Cuff Tear Arthropathy with Different Types of Shoulder Prostheses: Clinical Results (Median Constant Score, Age- and Sex-Corrected) Correlated with the Author's Classification System

Prosthesis	Type Ia	Type Ib	Type IIa	Type IIb
Conventional prosthesis	80 (5)	80 (4)	70 (3)	
Bipolar prosthesis		74 (3)	59 (3)	
Reversed prosthesis	91 (7)		92 (16)	90 (23)

In addition to age, the clinical presentation is also a very important factor in decision-making. If pain-related functional impairment is excluded, a conventional shoulder hemiarthroplasty would be unsuccessful in the prosthetic treatment of a highly pseudoparalytic shoulder—a shoulder with active flexion or abduction significantly lower than 90 degrees with the typical aspect of anterosuperior dislocation (**Fig. 3–9**). The clinical outcome would be some pain relief at best, with a highly unsatisfactory functional result. To offer these patients a satisfactory functional outcome, the only choice of prosthetic therapy is a reversed shoulder arthroplasty.

In younger patients, alternative therapies should be considered. Because of the extraanatomic design of the current reverse shoulder systems, there are mechanical disadvantages, mainly early glenoid component loosening or midterm inferior glenoid erosion, polyethylene-liner wear, and secondary midterm loosening of glenoid component. Therefore, younger patients with CTA should not be treated with a reverse shoulder arthroplasty. A conventional hemiarthroplasty, perhaps with some soft tissue reconstruction, may be considered. The decisive question in the preoperative decision-making relates to the biomechanical competence of the residual RC tear. This is determined by the RC's functional performance and by the radiological changes in the position of the center of rotation of the glenohumeral joint. Another decisive parameter is the quality and quantity of morphologic changes of the joint. The occurrence and presentation of the typical morphologic features of CTA is multifactorial and mainly dependent on the underlying pathology and the pathomechanics of the RC tear. The pathomechanics of the RC tear is highly dependent on the size and location of the tear, the number of tendons involved, the integrity of the coracoacromial arch, and the bony geometry of the glenoid.

Besides the clinical parameters (pseudoparalysis, lag signs), our radiological classification focusing on the position and stability of the center of rotation of the glenohumeral joint is a helpful tool in decision making for the type of prosthesis in CTA—especially in younger patients.

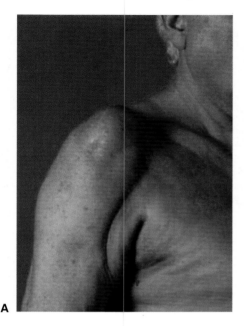
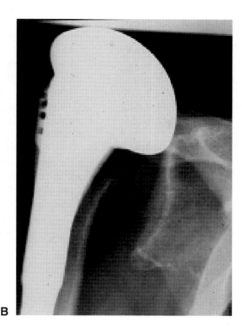

A   **B**

Figure 3–9 Typical (A) clinical and (B) radiologic appearance of a rotator cuff tear arthropathy with a biomechanically decompensated massive rotator cuff tear.

References

1. Nové-Josserand L, Levigne C, Noel E, Walch G. The acromiohumeral interval. A study of the factors influencing its height. Rev Chir Orthop Reparatrice Appar Mot 1996;82(7):608–614

2. Thomazeau H, Boukobza E, Morcet N, Chaperon J, Langlais F. Prediction of rotator cuff repair results by magnetic resonance imaging. Clin Orthop Relat Res 1997;344:275–288

3. Goutallier D, Postel JM, Lavau L, et al. Impact of fatty degeneration of the supraspinatus and infraspinatus muscles on the prognosis of surgical repair of the rotator cuff. Rev Chir Orthop Reparatrice Appar Mot 1999;85:668–676

4. Thompson WO, Debski RE, Boardman ND III, et al. A biomechanical analysis of rotator cuff deficiency in a cadaveric model. Am J Sports Med 1996;24(3):286–292

5. Grammont PM, Baulot E. Delta shoulder prosthesis for rotator cuff rupture. Orthopedics 1993;16:65–68

6. De Wilde L, Audenaert E, Barbaix E, Audenaert A, Soudan K. Consequences of deltoid muscle elongation on deltoid muscle performance: a computerized study. Clin Biomech (Bristol, Avon) 2002;17(7):499–505

7. Lee SB, Kim KJ, O'Driscoll SW, Morrey BF, An KN. Dynamic glenohumeral stability provided by the rotator cuff muscles in the midrange and end-range of motion. A study in cadavera. J Bone Joint Surg Am 2000;82(6):849–857

8. Hsu HC, Boardman ND III, Luo ZP, An KN. Tendon-defect and muscle-unloaded models for relating a rotator cuff tear to glenohumeral stability. J Orthop Res 2000;18(6):952–958

9. Sharkey NA, Marder RA. The rotator cuff opposes superior translation of the humeral head. Am J Sports Med 1995;23(3):270–275

10. Yamaguchi K, SherJ S, Andersen WK, et al. Glenohumeral motion in patients with rotator cuff tears: a comparison of asymptomatic and symptomatic shoulders. J Shoulder Elbow Surg 2000;9(1):6–11

11. Parsons IM, Apreleva M, Fu FH, Woo SL. The effect of rotator cuff tears on reaction forces at the glenohumeral joint. J Orthop Res 2002;20(3):439–446

12. Kido T, Itoi E, Konno N, Sano A, Urayama M, Sato K. The depressor function of biceps on the head of the humerus in shoulders with tears of the rotator cuff. J Bone Joint Surg Br 2000;82(3):416–419

13. Rittmeister M, Kerschbaumer F. Grammont reverse total shoulder arthroplasty in patients with rheumatoid arthritis and nonreconstructible rotator cuff lesions. J Shoulder Elbow Surg 2001;10:17–22

14. Neer CS 2nd, Craig EV, Fukuda H. Cuff-tear arthropathy. J Bone Joint Surg Am 1983;65(9):1232–1244

15. McCarty DJ, Halverson PB, Carrera GF, Brewer BJ, Kozin F. "Milwaukee shoulder"–association of microspheroids containing hydroxyapatite crystals, active collagenase, and neutral protease with rotator cuff defects. I. Clinical aspects. Arthritis Rheum 1981;24(3):464–473

16. Neer CS. Shoulder Reconstruction. Philadelphia, PA: WB Saunders, 1990:143–272, 405–406

17. Lehtinen JT, Kaarela K, Belt EA, Kautiainen HJ, Kauppi MJ, Lehto M. Relation of glenohumeral and acromioclavicular joint destruction in rheumatoid shoulder. A 15 year follow up study. Ann Rheum Dis 2000;59(2):158–160

18. Hamada K, Fukuda H, Mikasa M, Kobayashi Y. Roentgenographic findings in massive rotator cuff tears. A long term observation. Clin Orthop 1990;254:92–96

19. Farvard L, Lautmann S, Clement P. Osteoarthritis with massive rotator cuff-tear. In: Walch G, Boileau P, eds. Shoulder Arthroplasty. Berlin-Heidelberg: Springer, 1999: 261–266

20. Burkhart SS. Fluoroscopic comparison of kinematic patterns in massive rotator cuff tears. A suspension bridge model. Clin Orthop 1992;284:144–152

21. Visotsky JJ, Basamania C, Seebauer L, Rockwood CA, Jensen KL. Cuff tear arthropathy: pathogenesis, classification, and algorithm for treatment. J Bone Joint Surg Am 2004; 86:35–40

22. Seebauer L, Walter W, Keyl W. Reverse total shoulder arthroplasty for the treatment of defect arthropathy. Oper Orthop Traumatol 2005;1:1–24

23. Seebauer L, Keyl W. Inverse Schulterprothese Delta3® n. Grammont - Differentialindikation und Frühergebnisse. Z Orthop 2001;139 (Suppl 1):85

24. Neer CS, Watson KC, Stanton FJ. Recent experience in total shoulder replacement. J Bone Joint Surg Am 1982;64:319–337

25. Wirth MA, Jensen KL. The effect of previous coraco-acromial arch surgery on the outcome of shoulder arthroplasty. Paper presented

at: 8th International Congress on Surgery of the Shoulder, April 23–26,2001; Cape Town, South Africa

26. Williams GR Jr, Rockwood CA Jr. Hemiarthroplasty in rotator cuff deficient shoulders. J Shoulder Elbow Surg 1996;5:362–367

27. Jensen KI, Williams GR Jr, Russell J, et al. Rotator cuff tear arthropathy. J Bone Joint Surg Am 1999;81:1312–1324

28. Post M, Jablon M. Constrained total shoulder arthroplasty. Long term follow-up observations. Clin Orthop Relat Res 1983;173:109–116

29. De Buttet M, Bouchon Y, Capon D, Delfosse J. Grammont shoulder arthroplasty for osteoarthritis with massive rotator cuff tears—report of 71 cases. J Shoulder Elbow Surg 1997;6:197

30. Vrettos BC, Wallace WA, Neumann L. Bipolar hemiarthroplasty of the shoulder for the elderly patient with rotator cuff arthropathy. J Bone Joint Surg Br 1998; 80(Suppl 1):106

31. Worland RL, Jessup DE, Arredondo J, Warburton KJ. Bipolar shoulder arthroplasty for rotator cuff arthropathy. J Shoulder Elbow Surg 1997;6:512–515

32. Constant CR, Murley AH. A clinical method of functional assessment of the shoulder. Clin Orthop Relat Res 1987;214:160–164

33. Sirveaux F, Farvard L, Oudet D, et al. Grammont inverted total shoulder arthroplasty in the treatment of glenohumeral osteoarthritis with massive rupture of the cuff. J Bone Joint Surg Br 2004;86:388–395

34. Frankle M, Siegal S, Pupello D, et al. The reverse shoulder prosthesis for glenohumeral arthritis associated with severe rotator cuff deficiency. A minimum two-year follow-up study of sixty patients. J Bone Joint Surg Am 2005;87:1697–1705

35. Farvard L. Guery J, Bicknell R, et al. Survivorship of the reverse prosthesis. In: Walch G, Boileau P, Mole D, et al., editors. Reverse Shoulder Arthroplasty—clinical results—complications—revisions. Montpelier, VT: Sauramps Medical, 2006;373–380

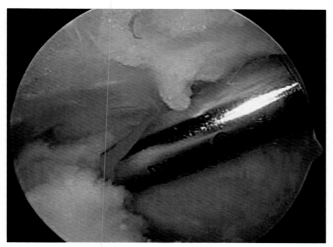

Figure 4–14 Arthroscopic image of the subdeltoid bursa being detached from the deltoid.

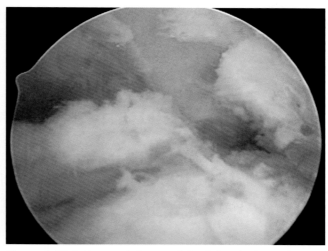

Figure 4–15 Arthroscopic image of the infraspinatus and supraspinatus interval; the spine of the scapula has been exposed.

should be approached anteriorly and the posteriorly. With the posterior interval release, the spine of the scapula is cleaned with the shaver and the capsular side of the RC is released. The interval is then released medially with an electrocautery or a shaver blade until the fat of the suprascapular nerve is exposed at the spinoglenoid notch (**Fig. 4–18**).

Arthroscopic Suprascapular Nerve Decompression

The mobility of a torn RC has significant importance when attempting to repair it without undue tension. The suprascapular nerve has been shown to act as a cuff tether as it traverses under the transverse scapular ligament in the suprascapular notch (**Fig. 4–19**).[20] Additionally, studies have shown that tension is placed on the nerve when cuff retraction is present.[21] Some patients with massive RC tears have electromyogram (EMG) evidence of muscle denervation of the supraspinatus and infraspinatus muscles.[22] Some surgeons release the suprascapular nerve at the time of cuff mobilization in anticipation of repair and the hope of improved nerve and muscle recovery. The criteria for decompression include patients with documented EMG evidence of muscle denervation from suprascapular nerve compression.[23]

Arthroscopic suprascapular nerve decompression is performed with the arthroscope inserted through a modified posterolateral portal and a radiofrequency device from the

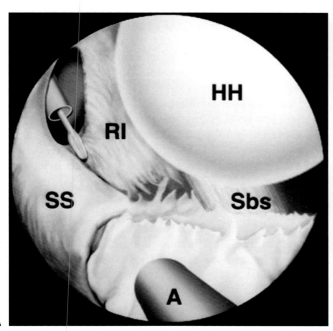

A

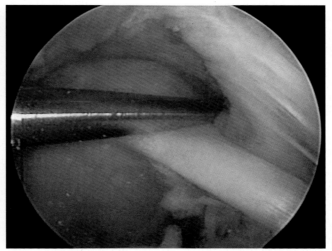

B

Figure 4–16 (A) Artist's rendering, and **(B)** arthroscopic image of the release of the coracohumeral ligament.

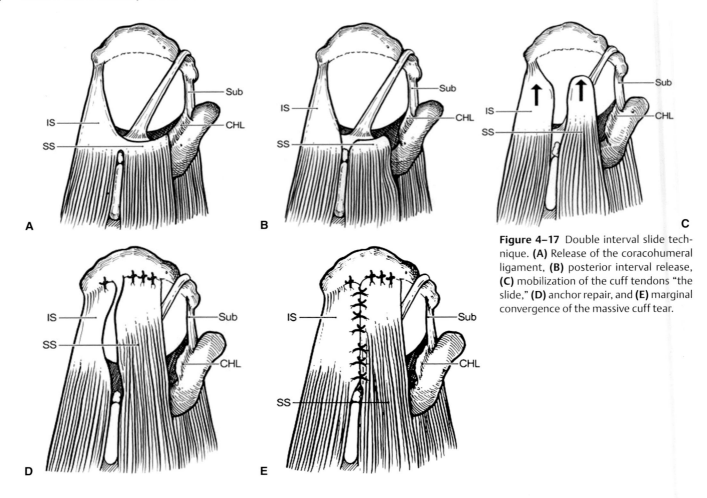

Figure 4–17 Double interval slide technique. **(A)** Release of the coracohumeral ligament, **(B)** posterior interval release, **(C)** mobilization of the cuff tendons "the slide," **(D)** anchor repair, and **(E)** marginal convergence of the massive cuff tear.

lateral portal.[23,24] By following the CA ligament anteroinferiorly, identification of the coracoid base and the transverse scapular ligament is facilitated.[12] A modified Neviaser portal is then utilized for probe placement and subsequent transverse scapular ligament release. Release of the ligament is more safely performed on the lateral side of the suprascapular notch via subperiosteal elevation from the coracoid base. This can be performed with a radiofrequency device, beaver blade, or curved electrocautery (**Fig. 4–20**).[23]

Rotator Cuff Repair after Appropriate Mobilization

Upon introduction of the scope into the subacromial space proper delineation of the tear configuration must be performed. This is facilitated by an adequate bursectomy and placement of the scope in more than one portal to allow for spatial awareness. Advancement of the RC to the properly prepared bony footprint of the greater tuberosity should be attempted with a grasper (**Fig. 4–21A-C**). Undue tension on the repair should be avoided due to subsequent cuff fail-

ure occurring. If adequate lateralization of the cuff cannot be done, then the footprint may be medialized 5 to 10 mm (**Fig. 4–21D**).[25] Additionally, advancement of the supraspinatus and infraspinatus can be performed via interval slides to enable proper repair. CR proceeds in a sequential fashion starting with advancement of the infraspinatus anteriorly and laterally followed by "marginal convergence" if necessary and completed with supraspinatus lateralization. Marginal convergence involves the placement of sutures between the supraspinatus and infraspinatus tendons or between the supraspinatus and biceps tendon and functions to reduce the tension on the tendon to footprint reconstruction.[26–39] The first double loaded suture anchor is placed near the articular surface and the cuff is initially secured with a mattress stitch. The second suture pair from the anchor is then placed in a "T-type" mattress locking stitch (**Fig. 4–22**). Additional suture anchors are placed in single file as needed along the articular margin. Recent literature has focused on double-row suture anchor RC repair.[27–43] Studies have shown that greater surface area contact with the footprint is achieved initially.[28,29] Whether or not this is important in repair healing has not been proven

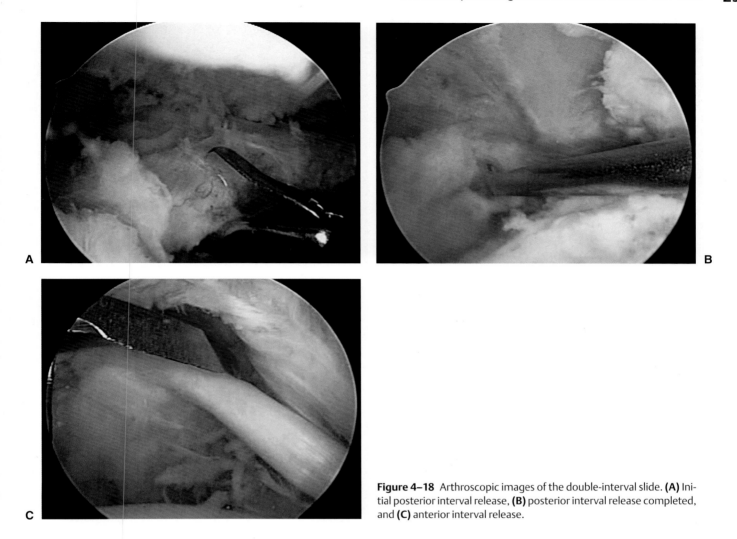

Figure 4–18 Arthroscopic images of the double-interval slide. **(A)** Initial posterior interval release, **(B)** posterior interval release completed, and **(C)** anterior interval release.

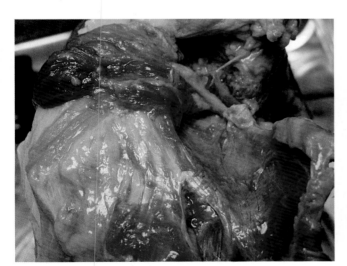

Figure 4–19 Cadaveric suprascapular nerve release.

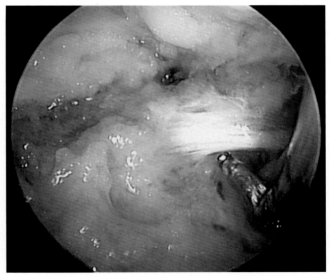

Figure 4–20 Arthroscopic image of decompression of the suprascapular nerve.

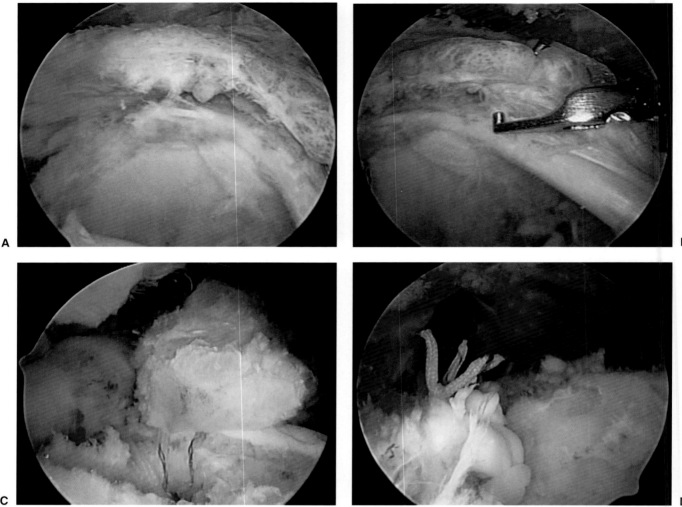

Figure 4–21 Arthroscopic image showing mobilization of the supraspinatus and infraspinatus tendons anterolaterally. **(A)** Before mobilization, **(B)** mobilization with a grasper, **(C)** after mobilization with suture placement, and **(D)** medialization of the rotator cuff footprint to achieve a proper tension repair.

clinically. If lateral uplifting of the repair occurs after medial anchor placement, placement of a second suture anchor more laterally on the footprint or tuberosity serves to reduce this tissue (**Fig. 4–23A**).

For massive cuff repairs, we prefer metal, dual-loaded suture anchors (Smith & Nephew Twin-Fix; Smith & Nephew, Inc., Andover, MA, or equivalent), high-strength sutures (Smith & Nephew Ultra Braid or equivalent), and an interlocking suture, such as the T-suture, mattress equivalent.[30,31] Newer anchors with improved bone holding and high-strength sutures have now made the tendon suture interface the weak link in the repair. The strongest bone for suture anchor purchase is either just medial to the articular margin and under the articular surface or laterally on the greater tuberosity. Typical patients with massive cuff tears tend to have an osteoporotic lateral footprint; hence they do not hold suture anchors well. Recessed suture eyelets with peripheral cortical purchase by the anchor may

very well solve this dilemma. For suture passage through tendon, we prefer a direct suture passing technique (Smith & Nephew E-pass), a retrograde pierce and grab technique (**Fig. 4–23B**) (Smith & Nephew Arthro pierce), or suture shuttle technique (Smith & Nephew Accupass).

Tissue Repair Enhancement

As science progresses, advancements in tissue repair enhancement abound. Techniques for enhancing a cuff repair include bursal augmentation of the repair, growth factor placement, and pulsed ultrasound. Uhthoff et al[32] has written extensively on the subacromial bursa as an important source of pluripotent cells for repair. The bursal tissue, in fact, does have an extensive vascular network and has been referred to as the bursal epoetin. Whether or not these cells are the actual initiators or enhancers of cuff tis-

7. Burkhart SS. Fluoroscopic comparison of kinematic patterns in massive rotator cuff tears. A suspension bridge model. Clin Orthop Relat Res 1992; 284:144–152

8. Burkhart SS. Arthroscopic treatment of massive rotator cuff tears. Clinical results and biomechanical rationale. Clin Orthop Relat Res 1991;267:45–56

9. Ekin A, Ozcan C. Massive rotator cuff tears: diagnosis and treatment techniques. Acta Orthop Traumatol Turc 2003;37:87–92

10. Boileau P, Brassart N, Watkinson DJ, Carles M, Hatzidakis AM, Krishnan SG. Arthroscopic repair of full-thickness tears of the supraspinatus: does the tendon really heal? J Bone Joint Surg Am 2005;87(6):1229–1240

11. Goutallier D, Postel JM, Gleyze P, Leguilloux P, Van Driessche S. Influence of cuff muscle fatty degeneration on anatomic and functional outcomes after simple suture of full-thickness tears. J Shoulder Elbow Surg 2003;12(6):550–554

12. Lafosse L. Personal communication. Mitek Sports Fellowship Course. Colorado Springs, Jan. 6, 2006

13. Klinger HM, Spahn G, Baums MH, Steckel H. Arthroscopic debridement of irreparable massive rotator cuff tears–a comparison of debridement alone and combined procedure with biceps tenotomy. Acta Chir Belg 2005;105(3):297–301

14. Duralde XA, Bair B. Massive rotator cuff tears: the result of partial rotator cuff repair. J Shoulder Elbow Surg 2005;14(2):121–127

15. Burkhart SS. Partial repair of massive rotator cuff tears: the evolution of a concept. Orthop Clin North Am 1997;28:125–132

16. Matsen, FA III. The shoulder. In: Rockwood CA Jr., Matsen FA III, eds. 2nd ed. Philadelphia, PA: WB Saunders, 1998

17. Tauro JC. Arthroscopic "interval slide" in the repair of large rotator cuff tears. Arthroscopy 1999;15(5):527–530

18. Tauro JC. Arthroscopic repair of large rotator cuff tears using the interval slide technique. Arthroscopy 2004;20(1):13–21

19. Klein JR, Burkhart SS. Identification of essential anatomic landmarks in performing arthroscopic single- and double-interval slides. Arthroscopy 2004;20(7):765–770

20. Warner JP, Krushell RJ, Masquelet A, Gerber C. Anatomy and relationships of the suprascapular nerve: anatomical constraints to mobilization of the suprascapular and infraspinatus muscles in the management of massive rotator-cuff tears. J Bone Joint Surg Am 1992;74:36–45

21. Albritton MJ, Graham RD, Richards RS II, Basamania CJ. An anatomic study of the effects on the suprascapular nerve due to retraction of the supraspinatus muscle after a rotator cuff tear. J Shoulder Elbow Surg 2003;12:497–500

22. Hoellrich RG, Gasser SI, Morrison DS, Kurzweil PR. Electromyographic evaluation after primary repair of massive rotator cuff tears. J Shoulder Elbow Surg 2005;14(3):269–272

23. Lafosse L, Tomasi A. Technique for endoscopic release of suprascapular nerve entrapment at the suprascapular notch. Tech Shoulder Elbow Surg 2006;7(1):1–6

24. Lewicky YM, Dembitsky NPL, Patil S, Hoenecke H, Esch JC. Arthroscopic suprascapular nerve decompression: navigating to the transverse scapular ligament. Forthcoming

25. Liu J, Hughes RE, O'Driscoll SW, An KN. Biomechanical effect of medial advancement of the supraspinatus tendon. A study in cadavera. J Bone Joint Surg Am 1998;80:853–859

26. Burkhart SS, Danaceau SM, Pearce CE Jr. Arthroscopic rotator cuff repair: analysis of results by tear size and by repair technique–margin convergence versus direct tendon-to-bone repair. Arthroscopy 2001;17(9):905–912

27. LoI KY, Burkhart SS. Double-row arthroscopic rotator cuff repair: re-establishing the footprint of the rotator cuff. Arthroscopy 2003; 19:1035–1042

28. Tuoheti Y, Itoi E, Yamamoto N, et al. Contact area, contact pressure, and pressure patterns of the tendon-bone interface after rotator cuff repair. Am J Sports Med 2005;33:1869–1874

29. Kim DH, ElAttrache NS, Tibone JE, et al. Biomechanical comparison of a single-row versus double-row suture anchor technique for rotator cuff repair. Am J Sports Med 2006;34:1–8

30. Ma CB, MacGillivray JD, Clabeaux J, Lee S, Otis JC. Biomechanical evaluation of arthroscopic rotator cuff stitches. J Bone Joint Surg Am 2004;86-A(6):1211–1216

31. MacGillivray JD, Ma CB. An arthroscopic stitch for massive rotator cuff tears: the Mac stitch. Arthroscopy 2004;20(6):669–671

32. Uhthoff HK, Sano H, Trudel G, Ishii H. Early reactions after reimplantation of the tendon of supraspinatus into bone a study in rabbits. J Bone Joint Surg Br 2000;82-B:1072–1076

33. Montenegro S. Personal communication, 2005.

34. Koeke PU, Parizotto NA, Carrinho PM, Salate AC. Comparative study of the efficacy of the topical application of hydrocortisone, therapeutic ultrasound and phonophoresis on the tissue repair process in rat tendons. Ultrasound Med Biol 2005;31: 345–350

35. Warden SJ. A new direction for ultrasound therapy in sports medicine. Sports Med 2003;33(2):95–107

36. Ballantyne BT, O'Hare SJ, Paschall JL, et al. Electromyographic activity of selected shoulder muscles in commonly used therapeutic exercises. Phys Ther 1993;73:668–677

37. Audenaert E, Van Nuffel J, Schepens A, Verhelst M, Verdonk R. Reconstruction of massive rotator cuff lesions with a synthetic interposition graft: a prospective study of 41 patients. Knee Surg Sports Traumatol Arthrosc 2006; 14(4):360–364

38. Sclamberg SG, Tibone JE, Itamura JM, Kasraeian S. Six-month magnetic resonance imaging follow-up of large and massive rotator cuff repairs reinforced with porcine small intestinal submucosa. J Shoulder Elbow Surg 2004;13(5):538–541

39. Sharkey NA, Marder RA. The rotator cuff opposes superior translation of the humeral head. Am J Sports Med 1995;23(3):270–275

40. Bittar ES. Arthroscopic management of massive rotator cuff tears. Arthroscopy 2002;18:104–106

41. Burkhart SS. Arthroscopic treatment of massive rotator cuff tears. Clin Orthop Relat Res 2001;390:107–118

42. Galatz LM, Ball CM, Teefey SA, Middleton WD, Yamaguchi K. The outcome and repair integrity of completely arthroscopically repaired large and massive rotator cuff tears. J Bone Joint Surg Am 2004;86-A(2):219–224

43. Jones CK, Savoie FH III. Arthroscopic repair of large and massive rotator cuff tears. Arthroscopy 2003;19(6):564–571

44. Sperling JW, Cofield RH, Schleck C. Rotator cuff repair in patients fifty years of age and younger. J Bone Joint Surg Am 2004;86-A(10):2212–2215

45. Tashjian RZ, Henn RF, Kang L, Green A. The effect of comorbidity on self-assessed function in patients with a chronic rotator cuff tear. J Bone Joint Surg Am 2004;86-A(2):355–362

46. Vad VB, Warren RF, Altchek DW, O'Brien SJ, Rose HA, Wickiewicz TL. Negative prognostic factors in managing massive rotator cuff tears. Clin J Sport Med 2002;12(3):151–157

47. Tokish JM, Decker MJ, Ellis HB, Torry MR, Hawkins RJ. The belly-press test for the physical examination of the subscapularis muscle: electromyographic validation and comparison to the lift-off test. J Shoulder Elbow Surg 2003;12(5):427–430

48. Walch G, Boulahia A, Calderone S, Robinson AH. The 'dropping' and 'hornblower's' signs in evaluation of rotator-cuff tears. J Bone Joint Surg Br 1998;80(4):624–628

49. LoI K, Burkhart SS. Arthroscopic repair of massive, contracted, immobile rotator cuff tears using single and double interval slides: technique and preliminary results. Arthroscopy 2004;20:22–33

50. LoI K, Burkhart SS. The interval slide in continuity: a method of mobilizing the anterosuperior rotator cuff without disrupting the tear margins. Arthroscopy 2004;20:435–441

51. Burkhart SS. The principle of margin convergence in rotator cuff repair as a means of strain reduction at the tear margin. Ann Biomed Eng 2004;32(1):166–170

52. Richards DP, Burkhart SS. Margin convergence of the posterior rotator cuff to the biceps tendon. Arthroscopy 2004;20(7):771–775

53. Mazzocca AD, Millett PJ, Guanche CA, Santangelo SA, Arciero RA. Arthroscopic single-row versus double-row suture anchor rotator cuff repair. Am J Sports Med 2005;33:1–8

54. Dockery ML, Wright TW, LaStayo PC. Electromyography of the shoulder: an analysis of passive modes of exercise. Orthopedics 1998;21(11):1181–1184

55. Hintermeister RA, Lange GW, Schultheis JM, Bey MJ, Hawkins RJ. Electromyographic activity and applied load during shoulder rehabilitation exercises using elastic resistance. Am J Sports Med 1998;26(2):210–220

56. McCann PD, Wootten ME, Kadaba MP, Bigliani LU. A kinematic and electromyographic study of shoulder rehabilitation exercises. Clin Orthop Relat Res 1993; 288:179–188

57. McMahon PJ, Debski RE, Thompson WO, Warner JJ, Fu FH, Woo SL. Shoulder muscle forces and tendon excursions during glenohumeral abduction in the scapular plane. J Shoulder Elbow Surg 1995;4(3):199–208

58. Roe C, Brox JI, Saugen E, Vollestad NK. Muscle activation in the contralateral passive shoulder during isometric shoulder abduction in patients with unilateral shoulder pain. J Electromyogr Kinesiol 2000;10(2):69–77

59. Smith J, Padgett DJ, Dahm DL, et al. Electromyographic activity in the immobilized shoulder girdle musculature during contralateral upper limb movements. J Shoulder Elbow Surg 2004;13(6):583–588

60. Wise MB, Uhl TL, Mattacola CG, Nitz AJ, Kibler WB. The effect of limb support on muscle activation during shoulder exercises. J Shoulder Elbow Surg 2004;13(6):614–620

61. Moore DR, Cain EL, Schwartz ML, Clancy WG Jr. Allograft reconstruction for massive, irreparable rotator cuff tears. Am J Sports Med 2006;34(3):392–396

62. Mura N, O'Driscoll SW, Zobitz ME, Heers G, An KN. Biomechanical effect of patch graft for large rotator cuff tears: a cadaver study. Clin Orthop Relat Res 2003; 415:131–138

63. Seldes RM, Abramchayev I. Arthroscopic insertion of a biologic rotator cuff tissue augmentation after rotator cuff repair. Arthroscopy 2006;22(1):113–116

5 Muscle Transfers for the Treatment of the Irreparable Rotator Cuff Tear

Robert C. Decker and Spero G. Karas

The main goals in rotator cuff (RC) repair are to establish continuity of the tendon, restore the soft tissue interface with the overlying acromion, center the humeral head in the glenoid, and relieve impingement.[1] Failure of these goals and failure to achieve repair of the RC is thought to lead to the development of cuff tear arthropathy. A loss of normal humeral head depression, which is supplied by a balanced RC unit, results in the upward migration of the humeral head. This, in turn, alters the force vector across the glenohumeral joint, leading to early degenerative changes. Additionally, with massive RC tear the humeral head is not effectively stabilized in the anterior and posterior direction, resulting in additional abnormal sheer forces compounding the abnormal wear pattern.[2]

RC tear repair, in general, has demonstrated good long-term results with clinical improvements.[2-10] Outcomes of repair correspond to the size or the RC tear, with massive tears presenting the most difficult surgical challenge.[6,10,11] No universally agreed upon definition or treatment of a massive RC tear has been established. Cofield[3] defined massive as any tear with a diameter >5 cm. Others have defined a massive tear as those tears involving at least two tendons.[4] Intraoperatively, two findings are important in determining if the massive RC tear is repairable: the elasticity of the muscle and the assessment of the possibility of direct tendon reinsertion into bone after excision of the necrotic ends.[5] Most large or massive RC tears are repairable; however, 5% of all RC tears are mechanically irreparable.[6] Additionally, the repair of chronic, retracted tears involving two or more tendons is technically difficult and has been shown to be less successful.[7-10]

In those instances where mobilization and direct repair of tendons is unattainable or has failed, an additional procedure may be required. Adequate results have been obtained from simple débridement and decompression of massive RC tears and partial repairs.[11,12] If débridement proves unsuccessful, then transfer of local tissues may be required to alleviate pain and improve function. Many tendon transfer techniques have been described for the management of massive, irreparable RC tear. These include mobilization of the superior cuff and transposition of the long head of the biceps tendon,[11,13] supraspinatus muscle advancement,[14-22] latissimus dorsi transfer,[4,15-26] subscapularis transfer,[3,16] trapezius transfer,[17-31] teres major transfer,[18-34] pectoralis major transfer,[19] teres minor transfer,[1]

combined subscapularis and teres minor,[20] and the deltoid muscle flap.[21,22] Although numerous techniques have been illustrated, no gold standard exists yet. The multitude of different transfers and the variability in the results of these techniques demonstrates a general lack of consensus on optimal treatment. Within this chapter, we will explore the most commonly described tendon transfer techniques, their indications, contraindications, and results.

It is important to understand the pathology present within the shoulder prior to surgery. This information should be sought preoperatively with plain radiographs in orthogonal planes, magnetic resonance imaging (MRI), and a thorough clinical exam. Muscle wasting in the supraspinatus fossa, weakness of external rotation (ER), and abnormal scapulothoracic motion should alert the clinician to the potential for a massive RC tear.[23] Additionally, it is important to know the main complaint of the patient, their functional status, and expectations from reconstructive surgery. Armed with this information the surgeon can best plan which reconstructive procedure to utilize.

Subscapularis Transfer

Subscapularis transfer is used for massive RC tears that cannot be primarily repaired. Because this transfer has been associated with diminished active elevation postoperatively, it is best performed on those unable to elevate the extremity above their head or in whom overhead function is markedly impaired.[24] Additionally, the patient should have a subscapularis amenable to mobilization. Therefore, the ideal patient for subscapularis transfer has a massive tear that is not amenable to primary fixation, cannot elevate the arm, and has an adequate subscapularis musculotendinous unit.

Surgical Technique

Cofield[3] first described the subscapularis transfer in 1982 for patients with tendon deficiency preventing primary repair. Through an anterior deltoid approach, the deltoid is elevated from the anterior acromion with care to provide a good sleeve for repair. An anterior acromioplasty is performed with resection of the coracoacromial ligament and decompression of the subacromial space and supraspinatus outlet. A limited débridement is performed to obtain a good vascular edge for healing. The upper half to two thirds of the subscapularis is mobilized by incising the musculotendinous junction in an oblique manner downward and medially (**Fig. 5–1**). The subscapularis can be divided due to its dual innervation from the superior and inferior subscapular nerves. The distal half of the subscapularis is left intact as an important passive and dynamic stabilizer of the shoulder. Soft tissue attachments are detached, while protecting both the axillary and musculocutaneous nerves. The upper part of the subscapularis is advanced superiorly and laterally to a cancellous trough medial to the greater tuberosity. The free edge is secured into the cancellous trough and the trimmed bleeding edges of the supraspinatus and infraspinatus are sewn to the transferred subscapularis to close the defect (**Fig. 5–2**).

Finally, the shoulder is ranged to evaluate the repair and ensure that the transfer is not overtensioned.[24] Postoperative management requires closely supervised physical therapy. Intraoperative ROM should guide postoperative physical therapy. Passive ROM and pendulum exercises are initiated immediately to prevent adhesions or contractures. ER is avoided as the subscapularis is mobilized superiorly and will be put under tension. Active ROM is initiated at 6 weeks; ER is begun at 2 to 3 months.

In Cofield's[3] initial series of 29 patients, 10 underwent subscapularis transfer for degenerative RC disease. Half felt that they improved significantly, whereas the other half felt they were only slightly improved and the average postoperative active elevation was 130 degrees. RJ and TJ Neviaser[36] found that transfer of the subscapularis and teres minor was a good salvage procedure for a massive

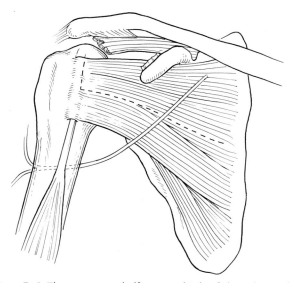

Figure 5–1 The upper one half to two thirds of the subscapularis is incised from its insertion on the lesser tuberosity. A bone trough is prepared for insertion of the transferred tendon onto the greater tuberosity.

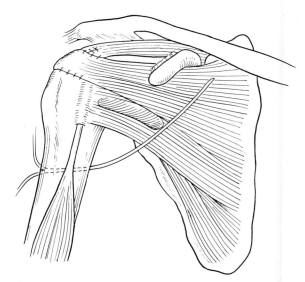

Figure 5–2 Completed subscapularis transfer. The medial edge of the transferred subscapularis tendon is sewed to the remnant lateral edge of the supraspinatus. Laterally, the subscapularis is attached to the greater tuberosity with suture anchors or transosseous sutures.

RC tear providing decreased pain and improved function if the deltoid was intact. They found deltoid dysfunction in three out of five failures. In 1983, Neer[25] described use of the upper 70% of the subscapularis for closure of large superior defects. In a series of 33 patients followed for a mean of 4.5 years, 16 had excellent results while 9 were satisfied and 9 were unsatisfied. The unsatisfied group primarily complained of decreased strength. Karas[16] felt caution should be utilized in selecting patients to undergo subscapularis transfer due to the potential for loss of function. In a retrospective review of 20 patients who underwent subscapularis transfer and subacromial decompression for massive, irreparable RC tears, Karas noted that 17 out of 20 patients were satisfied at a mean of 30 months. Nineteen described a decrease in pain postoperatively; 9 patients still had weakness and pain with prolonged overhead activities. Two patients lost active elevation despite reduction in pain and felt that the operation made them worse—possibly due to the loss of stabilization of the humeral head.[16,24] The transfer provides excellent pain relief, but caution should be exercised in doing this transfer in patients who have intact overhead function because this has been shown to potentially deteriorate.[16,24]

Subscapularis transfer is not without potential complications. The subscapularis acts as a humeral head depressor due to its insertional relationship into the lesser tuberosity. With transfer of the proximal half to two thirds of the subscapularis, there might not be enough force to depress the head actively, while the deltoid elevates the arm. With the subscapularis transferred superiorly, the anterior force vector may not be able to balance the posterior force vector. Additional potential complications include injury to the musculocutaneous nerve and the axillary nerve as it crosses the subscapularis. An additional theoretical complication is anterior instability resulting from transferring the upper half to two thirds of the subscapularis superiorly leaving only the lower third intact. While mobilizing the subscapularis, it is important not to violate the anterior capsule to protect against anterior instability.

Overall, subscapularis transfer is a useful procedure when the RC cannot be closed by conventional methods. However, the surgeon should be aware of the potential loss of forward elevation after subscapularis transfer. Furthermore, subscapularis transfer violates what is often the only intact, functioning, major muscle unit in patients with massive RC tear. Healing complications or rupture of the transferred muscle unit may result in no intact muscle group about the glenohumeral joint. For this reason, subscapularis transfer should likely not be the first choice in one's armamentarium for muscle transfer in massive RC tear.

Latissimus Dorsi

The latissimus dorsi transfer was conceived to allow closure of the RC defect with a vascularized, autogenous tendon, while providing head depressor activity and restoration of ER.[15] Originally a treatment for poliomyelitis and brachial plexus injuries, the transfer was intended to partially restore abduction as well as stabilization of the glenohumeral fulcrum.[26–45] The latissimus dorsi is a strong extrinsic internal rotator and adductor of the humerus, which receives its innervation from the thoracodorsal nerve and its vascular supply through the thoracodorsal pedicle lying on the anterolateral surface of the muscle. Saha[27] determined that the latissimus is active throughout shoulder ROM, so synergy with a new function is attainable with proper muscle retraining and rehabilitation.

Zachary[28] reported the first case of a latissimus dorsi transfer in a child with brachial plexopathy. He transferred both the latissimus and the teres major to the posterior humerus to improve ER. In 1988, Gilbert et al[29] and Gerber et al[30] reported on the technique of latissimus dorsi transfer for loss of ER and superior humeral head migration in patients with massive RC tears. A massive defect of the RC is biomechanically similar to motor loss of the suprascapular nerve, thus a latissimus dorsi transfer provides abduction, ER, and depressor forces to the glenohumeral joint. The primary indication for latissimus transfer is ER weakness due to loss of infraspinatus function. Pain and forward elevation loss are relative indications for latissimus transfer. Although not an absolute contraindication, Gerber et al noted that those patients with subscapularis insufficiency fared less well after latissimus dorsi transfer.

Surgical Technique

The patient is draped in the lateral decubitus position and a lateral incision across the axilla is utilized. The latissimus

dorsi is mobilized extensively along its superficial margins and mobilized off the scapula. The neurovascular pedicle is identified along the anteroinferior margin and protected along its course. The insertion of the latissimus dorsi is visualized by humeral abduction and internal rotation (IR). The tendon is then resected at its bony insertion. Care must be taken to avoid injuring the posterior humeral circumflex artery at the superior edge of the tendon. The radial nerve and axillary nerves are at risk during the tenotomy due to their proximity.[31–53] The tendon is mobilized to reach the posterosuperior aspect of the RC with the shoulder in 60 degrees of abduction. Not infrequently, the tendon may be short or thin, requiring augmentation with autogenous fascia lata. The tendon must track medial to the instant center of rotation of the shoulder joint throughout its arc of motion (**Fig. 5–3**). To maintain this path, the inferior enveloping fascia of the posterior deltoid may be used as a pulley. This will prevent lateral subluxation of the tendon; if it slips laterally it will become a primary adductor of the humerus. The tendon can then be sutured to the existing cuff tissue or used to close the defect as needed (**Fig. 5–4**). ROM is protected in an abduction brace for 6 to 8 weeks followed by gradual ROM and strengthening.

Gerber and colleagues[30] have demonstrated encouraging results with the latissimus dorsi transfer. They reported on 69 massive RC tears treated with latissimus dorsi transfer reviewed at an average of 53 months.[30] They found a significant improvement in pain, active flexion, active abduction, and active ER. Abduction strength also improved postoperatively. In this series, however, 13 patients with subscapularis insufficiency had minimal improvement in their postoperative outcome. The authors noted that the

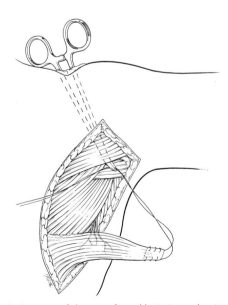

Figure 5–3 Passage of the transferred latissimus dorsi tendon deep to the posterior deltoid. The fascia of the posterior deltoid may be used as a "sling" to maintain a medial orientation of the tendon to the glenohumeral joint's instant center of rotation.

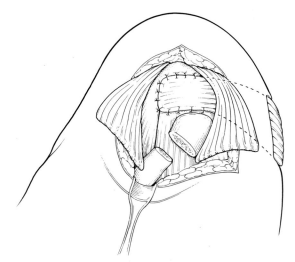

Figure 5–4 Attachment of the transferred latissimus dorsi tendon to the humeral head. When possible, the distal edge of the tendon should be attached to the superior aspect of the subscapularis tendon. Medially, the tendon is sewn to the remnant rotator cuff. Laterally, suture anchors or transosseous sutures are utilized to attach the latissimus tendon to the greater tuberosity.

procedure may be of limited benefit to those patients with a positive lift-off test preoperatively.

Aoki et al[32] prospectively reported on 12 shoulders that underwent latissimus dorsi transfer for irreparable cuff defects. Good to excellent results were found in eight cases, fair in one case, and poor in three cases. Function and pain were significantly improved. The mean postoperative active forward flexion was 135 degrees, which represented a 36-degree improvement from mean preoperative measurements. Osteoarthritic changes appeared in five shoulders and proximal migration of the humeral head occurred in six. Aoki and colleagues theorized that these changes occurred because the depressor action on the humeral head might not have been fully restored due to the latissimus dorsi not being fully active in the early phase of elevation. Electromyography revealed that 75% of transferred muscles showed synergistic action with the supraspinatus. Nonsynergistic motion was evident in three shoulders and was theorized to result from adhesions or rupture. Nonsynergy was associated with poor results. Risk factors for poor outcome were identified as multiple previous surgeries, deltoid pathology, and involvement of the subscapularis in the cuff defect.[32]

Miniacci and MacLeod[33] retrospectively reviewed 17 patients who were treated with a latissimus dorsi transfer for a massive RC tear. At a mean 51 months follow-up, 14 patients had significant pain relief and significant improvement in function for all activities except lifting more than 15 pounds. Fourteen stated they would have the operation again. Seven of 8 patients with a detached or nonfunctional anterior portion of the deltoid also had improvement. Interestingly, the authors of this series noted

that insufficiency of the subscapularis did not adversely affect postoperative outcome. There were three failures due to ongoing pain and impaired function. These 3 patients all had work-related injuries and viewed the operation as a failure. Warner and Parsons[34] evaluated the efficacy of primary transfer of the latissimus dorsi versus transfer as a salvage reconstruction for failed repairs. Salvage reconstruction of a failed prior RC repair yielded inferior results when compared with a primary latissimus dorsi transfer for irreparable RC tear. Warner and Parsons reviewed 16 patients who underwent transfer as salvage after a failed repair and 6 patients who underwent primary reconstruction. The salvage group had lower Constant scores (55 versus 70) and a higher rate of late rupture (44 versus 17%) compared with the primary group. Postoperative active forward flexion and ER were 122 degrees and 41 degrees in the primary group, with 105 degrees and 40 degrees in the salvage group, respectively. Inferior outcomes were found in patients with poor quality tendon, severe fatty degeneration, and deltoid detachment. Results of primary transfers in Warner and Parson's series were comparable to Gerber et al's series as 83% had good to excellent results. Lower gains were realized when utilized as a salvage procedure with only 50% reporting good to excellent results and 20% reporting poor outcomes. Warner and Parsons concluded that a competent deltoid is mandatory for the restoration of shoulder function once the tendon transfer achieves humeral head coverage. Patient selection is critical to this outcome. The authors noted that results similar to primary cases can be had with salvage only if the deltoid is intact.

Based on the encouraging results obtained by Gerber and others, the latissimus dorsi transfer has undergone increasing acceptance for posterosuperior tear configurations in patients that have limited ER and elevation with an intact subscapularis.

Pectoralis Major Transfer

Subscapularis tendon tears are rare and account for 3.5 to 8% of RC tears.[35,36] They are sometimes associated with anterior shoulder instability and respond poorly to nonoperative management.[35,37] Diagnosis is difficult and often causes a delay in treatment and a subsequently more-complex repair.[19,37–60] Gerber et al found that subscapularis tendons repaired early had better results than those with a delay to repair.[38] If left untreated, the subscapularis might not be amenable to repair due to retraction and atrophy. Pain may be accompanied by instability and abnormal glenohumeral kinematics.[39] Various transfers have been attempted for subscapularis tears, but the pectoralis major has had the most attention.[6,15,19,40–64]

Wirth and Rockwood originally described transferring the superior half of the pectoralis major tendon to the humeral head for reconstruction of a massive RC tear.[19] Resch et al[41] modified this transfer to approximate the natural course of the subscapularis more accurately.

Surgical Technique

Through a deltopectoral approach, the subscapularis, the conjoined tendon, tendon of the pectoralis major, and the anterior humeral head are all visualized. The long head of the biceps is tenotomized and tenodesed in those where it is dislocated anteriorly, and the superior half to two thirds of the pectoralis major is detached from the humerus and mobilized. Due to the segmental distribution of the thoracoacromial artery and pectoral nerve after passing under the clavicle, this does not compromise the neurovascular status of the pectoralis.[42] The musculocutaneous nerve and its entrance into the coracobrachialis muscle is identified and the space posterior to the conjoined tendon is developed. The pectoralis major tendon is then passed behind the conjoined tendon and anterior to the musculocutaneous nerve. Transosseous nonabsorbable sutures or suture anchors are utilized to attach the transferred pectoralis major (**Fig. 5–5**). If a partial or complete rupture of the supraspinatus is present, part of the pectoralis tendon is mobilized to the greater tuberosity to fill the defect. At the end of the procedure the musculocutaneous nerve is visualized to ensure that it is not under tension. The reconstructed shoulder is immobilized for 6 weeks. Passive ROM exercises are initiated on the day after surgery; after 6 weeks, active ROM is begun and full loading is allowed at 12 weeks.

Resch and colleagues[41] described their experience with 12 patients who had irreparable tears of the subscapula-

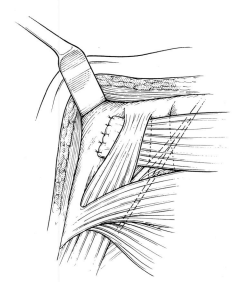

Figure 5–5 Completed pectoralis major transfer. The musculotendinous unit is mobilized and rerouted posterior to the conjoined tendon to reproduce the force vector of the subscapularis muscle. Care must be taken to identify and protect the musculocutaneous nerve.

ris tendon. They routed the transfer behind the conjoined tendon to the lesser tuberosity to reproduce the anatomy and biomechanics of the subscapularis. In their series, 8 patients had an isolated subscapularis tear; 4 patients had concomitant lesions of the supraspinatus. After a mean of 28 months, 9 patients subjectively reported excellent or good results, whereas 3 patients had fair results. No one had a poor subjective outcome. Pain decreased in all patients and Constant scores improved from an average of 22.6 points preoperatively to an average of 54.4 postoperatively. There was an increase in forward flexion from 93 degrees to 129 degrees and abduction improved from 85 degrees to 113 degrees. Resch et al also noted improved IR from the transfer; 3 patients with a preoperative positive "lift-off" test were negative postoperatively. Furthermore, 5 of 6 patients with positive "belly-press" tests preoperatively were negative after transfer. Electromyographic examination of the pectoralis major tendon demonstrated near symmetrical patterns of activity.[41]

Jost et al[40] evaluated 30 consecutive pectoralis muscle transfers for irreparable subscapularis tears with an average follow-up of 32 months. Unlike Resch and colleagues, Jost et al altered the transfer technique by transferring the entire pectoralis major muscle over the conjoined tendon. The transfer was fixed to the medial aspect of the greater tuberosity with bone anchors. Their technique was later modified to transosseous suture fixation secondary to insertion site pain in 11 of 18 shoulders. All 30 shoulders objectively were significantly improved. The Constant score increased from 47% preoperatively to 70% postoperatively, whereas shoulder subjective values improved from 23 to 55%. Pain, activities of daily living, forward flexion, and abduction strength all improved. Subjectively, 25 patients were either satisfied or very satisfied while 5 were either disappointed or dissatisfied. Outcome was determined to be less favorable when associated with an irreparable supraspinatus tear, and the transfer failed to restore full active anterior elevation.

Combined Pectoralis Major and Latissimus Dorsi Transfer

Building from earlier results on latissimus dorsi transfer for massive posterior cuff tears and pectoralis major transfers for anterior tears,[6,19] Aldridge et al[9] described a combined transfer for massive RC deficiency. Both the pectoralis major and latissimus dorsi were transferred to obtain a balanced fulcrum between the anterior and posterior forces of the cuff musculature.[2] The importance of the pectoralis transfer to the anterior defect was inferred from the results of Gerber and colleagues' earlier work on transferring the latissimus dorsi for posterior tears.[15,30,43] They found that patients who underwent latissimus dorsi transfer with a subscapularis tear failed to benefit from the transfer.[30]

Indications for a combined transfer include a massive RC deficiency, weakness, mild or no pain, and an inability to elevate the arm effectively at the GH joint. Patients with glenohumeral arthritis or a primary complaint of pain should, in general, be deemed poor candidates for tendon transfer.

Surgical Technique

The procedure combines elements of both the Sever-L'Episcopo procedure for brachial plexus birth palsies and the pectoralis major transfer for subscapularis defects.[19,34,44] Through a deltopectoral approach, the entire pectoralis major tendon and latissimus dorsi are removed from their insertions. The pectoralis major is transferred to the anterolateral superior humeral head and sutured to the superior aspect of the subscapularis tendon. Through a posterolateral incision the latissimus dorsi tendon is passed through the quadrilateral space inferior to the axillary nerve and posterior circumflex artery. The latissimus tendon is then fixed to the posterolateral superior humeral head and sutured to the remnants of the RC to close the posterior defect.[9] The latissimus dorsi is transferred for function only and no attempt is made to cover the entire humeral head. Patients are placed in an abduction brace for 6 weeks postoperatively, followed by a standard sling for 3 weeks. Passive and active assisted ROM and a strengthening program are instituted for a minimum of 3 months postoperatively.

Aldridge and colleagues retrospectively reviewed 11 patients with a combined transfer of the latissimus dorsi and pectoralis major tendon for massive RC deficiency. Patients' primary complaints were weakness and a decreased ability to elevate the affected arm. The primary preoperative objective was to improve function. Mean active elevation improved from 42 degrees preoperatively to 86 degrees postoperatively with mean ER improving from 2.3 degrees to 13 degrees. Overall, four patients made no improvement, two were slightly improved, and five improved significantly. The authors concluded that the combined procedure was an effective salvage technique to improve active elevation and ER in select patients with minimal pain who had failed both nonoperative and operative management. Indications on who would best benefit from this procedure are still being elucidated; nevertheless, it does hold promise for providing some patients with improved function.[9]

Triceps Transfer

Hartrampf et al[45] developed the triceps musculocutaneous flap as an alternative to the latissimus dorsi flap for chest wall reconstructions. Miller[46] used the triceps flap to cover large irreparable RC tears due to its ability to cover long distances. Malkani et al[47] investigated both the surgical anatomy of the long head of the triceps as well as prospectively evaluated their clinical experience in utilizing the long head of the triceps for reconstruction of massive RC tears. The authors felt that the transfer provided a vascularized space between the acromion and the humeral head to help alleviate pain. The primary indication for the triceps transfer was pain caused by supraspinatus and infraspinatus tears not amenable to repair.

Surgical Technique

The transfer procedure performed was originally described by Malkani and colleagues.[47] If the RC was irreparable, the muscular margins were débrided as necessary and transfer of the long head of the triceps was performed. The long head of the triceps was harvested through a long posterior humeral incision. The long head's tendon was divided roughly 1.5 cm above the olecranon process and the muscle was isolated to the level of its main pedicle (**Fig. 5–6**). The main pedicle was located roughly 2 to 3 cm distal to the teres major tendon. A tunnel was prepared by blunt dissection over the spine of the scapula to the subacromial space. The long head was then passed through the subacromial space mimicking the course of the infraspinatus. The transferred tendon was then attached to the humeral head and the remaining RC musculature (**Fig. 5–7**). A standardized rehabilitation program progressing from passive ROM to strengthening was instituted postoperatively.

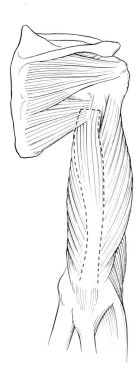

Figure 5–6 Area of mobilization for long head of triceps transfer. The tendon is taken down ~1.5 cm proximal to the olecranon process and mobilized to its main neurovascular pedicle ~3 cm distal to the teres minor.

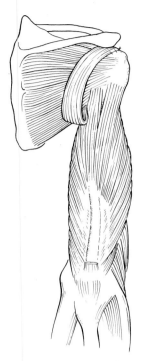

Figure 5–7 Completed triceps transfer. The tendon is routed deep to the posterior deltoid to replicate the course of the infraspinatus. The transferred tendon is subsequently attached to the greater tuberosity and the remnant rotator cuff tendons.

Malkani et al prospectively studied the 2-year clinical outcomes of triceps flap for coverage of irreparable RC tears. Nineteen transfers of the long head of the triceps transfer were evaluated in patients with massive, irreparable RC tears. All patients were subjectively satisfied with their outcome and had improvement in their pain, quality of life, and function. UCLA shoulder scores improved from 9.7 preoperatively to 28.8 postoperatively. Shoulder ROM improved in lateral rotation, ER, and forward elevation, while no difference was noted in abduction. Malkani and colleagues found no loss of elbow extension strength postoperatively from removing the long head of the triceps from the olecranon. This was consistent with Travill's[48] findings that the medial head of the triceps showed the greatest amount of activity with elbow extension and the long head the least amount of activity. Complications in Malkani et al's series included 1 patient who developed an ulnar neuropraxia and 2 patients had decreased sensation over the posterior arm postoperatively.[49]

In addition, Malkani and colleagues looked at 20 cadaver upper extremities to evaluate the surgical anatomy involved with long head of the triceps transfer. Entry points of neurovascular structures into the long head were measured from the distal margin of the teres major. An average of 3.2 important vascular pedicles was found, with the largest branch consistently located within 2 to 3 cm of the distal margin of the teres major tendon. Nerve branches from the radial nerve followed the vascular pedicles. The

average length of the long head of the triceps muscle was 24.4 cm from the distal margin of the teres major to the olecranon with an average width of 1.5 cm at its insertion. The authors noted that there was sufficient triceps to transfer to close a 5-cm defect in all cases.

Malkani et al felt that the triceps transfer did not suffer from the limitations of other transfers. These limitations include lack of sufficient flap to cover large defects, small range of advancement, and donor site morbidity. Additionally, the long head of the triceps flap is easily accessible in the standard shoulder surgery position and can be easily dissected without repositioning. The flap itself is extremely versatile and can be applied to several different configurations. Clinical results demonstrated decreased pain with improved function and quality of life. Primary indications should be for pain with massive defect and failure of repair in patients with low functional demands.

Teres Minor Transfer

In 1934, L'Episcopo described the first technique to rebalance the external and internal rotators in children with brachial plexus injuries using the teres minor.[44] A tendon to bone teres minor transfer had previously been described for treatment of RC tears.[1] Paavolainen modified this transfer by utilizing a bone block stabilized by internal fixation to provide increased fixation strength.[1] Indications for teres minor transfer are irreparable defects with badly frayed, contracted RC tendons of poor quality. In addition, as in most types of tendon transfer surgery, a cooperative patient is necessary due to the demanding nature of the long-term rehabilitation required.

Surgical Technique

The transfer is performed through an anterosuperior approach between the anterior and middle portions of the deltoid. First, the RC tendons are mobilized and evaluated for potential primary repair. Subacromial decompression of the bursa and acromioplasty are also completed at this time. If transfer is required, the arm is maximally internally rotated and the teres minor insertion is released with a block of cortico-cancellous bone. The capsule is released along the posterior glenoid rim to facilitate transfer of the muscle, tendon, and the capsule en bloc. The tendon, along with the bone block, is transferred anteriorly after removal of a similar-sized segment of bone from the site of the RC's previous insertion. The teres minor bone block, once in position, is secured with a cancellous screw. The bare bone block is then moved posteriorly and held in place by the RC so that no fixation is required (**Fig. 5–8**). Paavolainen felt a bone-to-bone interface allowed better healing capacity and longevity compared with previous tendon-to-bone reconstructions. With the size of the tear reduced,

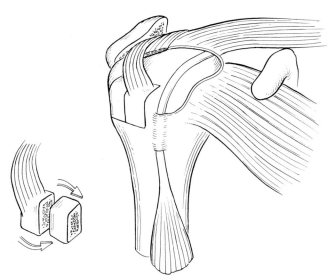

Figure 5–8 Teres minor tendon transfer. The teres minor is removed from the greater tuberosity with a bone block. A second bone block more anterior is removed to make room for the teres minor bone block and to fill the defect left from the teres minor harvest. The teres minor and its bone block are secured to the greater tuberosity with a screw and washer or transosseous sutures.

the remaining edges are sewn together. If a gap remains, an interval slide of the supraspinatus[50] or an advancement of the subscapularis[20] is performed. Passive exercises are initiated on the first postoperative day and continued for 6 weeks, at which time active exercises are begun. The cancellous screw is removed under local anesthesia 3 to 6 months postoperatively to prevent chronic impingement.[1]

Paavolainen[1] reported on 31 patients who underwent teres minor transfer for irreparable, massive RC tears. Night pain and activity-related pain improved in 93% of cases. In addition, he found that function in daily activities improved in 90% of patients. Although functional assessment scores were decreased in 3 patients, all patients were satisfied with relief of night pain.

In the setting of massive RC tear, glenohumeral force coupling is disrupted. The supraspinatus supplies 14% and the infraspinatus 22% of the force generation of the RC.[49] If this force coupling cannot be reestablished to normal, Paavolainen[1] felt transferring the teres minor was justified to improve function and relieve pain. The teres minor supplies 10% of the RC's normal force. In contrast, Karas[16] was reluctant to transfer the teres minor because of the possible weakening of abduction and ER.[51]

Paavolainen[1] felt that teres minor transfer was successful in pain relief when performed for the proper patient with a massive, irreparable RC defect. This transfer should be reserved for the patient with a badly frayed, retracted rupture and a retracted, poor quality tendon. Additionally, the patient should be able to comply fully with a long period of demanding rehabilitation. If these criteria are satis-

fied, teres minor transfer should provide pain relief and functional improvement.

Biceps Transfer Interposition Grafting

In 1975, Bush[13] first described biceps transfer interposition grafting (BTIG) as a means to close RC defects. He reported on 14 patients with limited follow-up and demonstrated good to excellent results in 75% of patients. The long head of the biceps was transferred into the tear after maximum mobilization of the RC to close down any residual defect. Pain was the primary indication for BTIG transfer. Additional indications were massive, irreparable RC tears with retraction and poor tissue; an intact long head of the biceps of good quality; a relatively normal glenohumeral joint; and a motivated patient able comply with therapy. Contraindications included paralysis of the remaining RC muscles or the deltoid, and degenerative changes in the glenohumeral joint.

Surgical Technique

Hansen[52] describes a modified Gardner incision from the anterolateral acromion to the lateral superior coracoid process. Subcutaneous flaps are elevated and the deltoid is split from the anterior acromion. Approximately 1 cm of deltoid is raised from the anterior acromion laterally and an anterior and inferior acromionectomy is performed. Alternatively, the arthroscope can be utilized to evaluate the RC tendon tear and the biceps tendon, decompress the bursa, and perform an acromioplasty and distal clavicle resection if necessary.

The anterior and posterior RC remnants are brought together and tension is restored. Where the cuff is insufficient to allow complete closure, BTIG is utilized to close the defect. The transverse ligament is incised and the biceps tendon is mobilized. A trough 1.5 cm posterior and lateral to the bicipital groove is made and the biceps tendon is mobilized into the groove. The tendon must be stable in both internal and ER in the new groove to maintain its normal function. The posterior RC remnant is then sutured to the posterior portion of the biceps and the anterior portion of the RC is sutured to the anterior portion of the biceps tendon. Remaining RC tissue is sutured to the bone to reinforce the repair (**Fig. 5–9**). Patients are placed in an abduction pillow postoperatively and pendulum exercises are instituted. A progressive rehabilitation program is sequentially instituted as healing ensues.[52]

Hansen[52] reported on 22 shoulders treated with BTIG followed for a minimum of 2 years. The primary indication for operative intervention was pain. Preoperatively, 19 of the 22 shoulders had significant rest pain, all but one had pain with use, and only one patient was able to sleep without difficulty. The average preoperative active elevation in

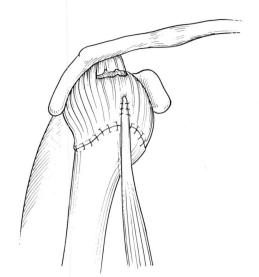

Figure 5–9 Biceps tendon interposition graft. The biceps tendon is mobilized and placed in an osseous trough 1.5 cm posterior to its native course. The remnant supraspinatus and infraspinatus are then mobilized and sewn to the biceps tendon. The repair is reinforced by sewing the remnant rotator cuff tendon edge to bone.

Deltoid Transfer

The deltoid muscular flap was described as a means to cover an exposed humeral head secondary to a RC defect. The transfer was initially described by Takagishi and later modified by Augereau and provides several advantages.[20,55,56] First, the insertion of a thick piece of tissue acts as a spacer between the humeral head and the acromion. Second, the deltoid flap remains contractile and vascularized. The contraction of the deltoid flap reinforces the action of the intrinsic and extrinsic depressor muscles of the humeral head, restoring scapulohumeral rhythm while permitting full active anterior elevation. During the first few degrees of active anterior elevation, the deltoid flap contracts concurrently with the deltoid. As the medial deltoid raises the humeral head, the contraction of the flap exerts a downward force on the humeral head. This will offset the elevating force of the deltoid during the first 60 degrees of active anterior elevation. The effectiveness of the deltoid flap is dependent on the quality of deltoid musculature. Therefore, a thin deltoid with signs of fatty degeneration is a contraindication to transfer.[21]

his series was 97 degrees. Additionally, none was able to perform all of the following activities of daily living: sleep, raising the arm, lifting 10 pounds, combing hair, or reaching the back pocket. Postoperatively, Hansen found that all patients were sleeping comfortably at night, 19 of 22 shoulders did not have rest pain, and all but two patients were able to perform all five aforementioned activities of daily living. Subjectively, all but one patient was pleased with their results and would have the procedure again. The only complication noted was a long head of the biceps rupture at 10 weeks postoperatively. The patient did not have any pain and was able to continue to perform all activities of daily living.[52]

Hansen stressed the importance of a complete and thorough subacromial decompression, as it was likely associated with significant pain relief.[53] The BTIG is not a replacement for RC tissue, but simply a vascularized, anchored graft allowing the reestablishment of the yoke mechanism between the anterior and posterior RC tendons. Therefore, a net resultant inferior head depressor effect can be reestablished. In addition, the graft is believed to help stabilize the humeral head and provide compression across the glenohumeral joint. Because the biceps is not sutured into its new groove, it remains a gliding tendon and maintains its original function as a humeral head stabilizer.[54] Hansen concluded that biceps tendon transfer does not result in additional harvest site morbidity and is a suitable technique to achieve cuff closure when unable to do so primarily. In those instances where standard techniques failed to close a massive tear, BTIG proved reliable and effective in improving function and relieving pain.

Surgical Technique

Gazielly[21] described an anterosuperior approach from the lateral clavicle passing over the acromioclavicular (AC) joint and finishing ~4 cm under the lateral edge of the acromion. The anterior deltoid is incised vertically along the axis of the AC joint to the junction between the middle and anterior heads of the deltoid. The lateral aspect of the anterior deltoid is then detached from the anterosuperior edge of the acromion subperiosteally to allow a firm cuff for repair. The anteromedial deltoid is left attached to the clavicle. If necessary, acromioplasty and decompression are performed if not previously performed during arthroscopic evaluation. The tear is then evaluated and resected back to a vascularized edge amenable to repair. The width of the flap needed depends on the width of the cuff tear in its sagittal plane. The base of the flap must be at least 2 to 3 cm to maintain vascularization and innervation. The flap is fashioned by cutting outward into the deltoid interval laterally and the previous performed deltoid incision medially (**Fig. 5–10**). Nonabsorbable sutures are passed first through the posterior segment of the tear and then passed through the leading edge of the deltoid flap. It is important to incorporate the deep deltoid fascia as a means to provide strength to the repair (**Fig. 5–11**). The deltoid defect is closed to help maintain shoulder contour and cosmesis postoperatively. A 70-degree-abduction sling and postoperative rehabilitation is started immediately. The two goals of rehabilitation are to protect the flap against subacromial compression and tensioning and to exercise the flap to maintain its contractile property and avoid atrophy.

Gazielly deemed postoperative exercise and therapy critical to success.[21]

Gazielly reviewed the outcomes of 20 patients treated for massive cuff tears with deltoid flap. All patients had failed a 6-month period of specific rehabilitation based on strengthening the humeral head depressor muscles. Additionally, all patients had full passive ROM preoperatively, as stiffness was a contraindication. All patients had pain and muscle weakness. Postoperatively, 45% of patients were free of pain and 55% had mild pain; postoperative level of activity was satisfactory in 65% of patients. Improvements were seen in active ROM, strength, and muscular fatigue. Results of Gazielly's series were similar to those obtained by Saragaglia and Tourne.[57] Results demonstrate that deltoid flap repair helped with pain and postoperative strength. Maximum strength was usually realized at 12 to 18 months postoperatively and patients were able to return to work as fatigue pain was relieved.[21]

Augereau reported on 22 deltoid flaps evaluated by MRI after 2.5 years and demonstrated 18 intact flaps. Results were better in those patients where the deltoid had a homogeneous stroma with a thickness of >2 mm after 2.5 years. Augereau reported 37% of humeral heads were centered postoperatively after deltoid transfer.[55] Gazielly followed his deltoid flaps with ultrasound and found 90% were intact at one year. No signs of impingement were found with intact transfers. Additionally, he found that flaps that were between 5 and 9 mm had excellent and good results, whereas flaps thinner than 4 mm did not do as well with four poor and one fair result. These results reinforced the need for a good quality deltoid for satisfactory transfer results.[22]

Deltoid transfer has been noted to be a reliable alternative for treating chronic, massive RC tears.[21,22] Deltoid transfer requires active, motivated adults with good deltoid muscle quality who have near normal active ROM, but suffer from pain and fatigue. Transfer is contraindicated in patients with signs of fatty muscular degeneration of the deltoid, as they have poorer postoperative results.

Trapezius Transfer

Mikasa and Yamanaka transferred the trapezius for RC defect coverage if the RC tendons could not be approximated to the greater tuberosity at 90 degrees of abduction at primary repair.[17–30,58] The trapezius is the largest of the suspensory muscles of the shoulder girdle and is divided into three parts: the upper, intermediate, and lower fibers. The upper and intermediate fibers were utilized for transfer. The upper fibers elevate the scapula along with the levator scapulae and the intermediate fibers adduct the scapula.

Surgical Technique

The lateral decubitus position is typically used to perform the trapezius transfer. A lateral incision is elongated to the medial border of the scapula ~1 cm superior to the spine of the scapula. The skin is mobilized to visualize the trapezius of which ~10 cm is detached from the spine of the scapula and 4 cm is detached from the distal clavicle. The acromial insertion is left untouched. About 8 cm of the trapezius is separated in parallel to its muscle fibers and the muscle belly is elevated. The insertion of the trapezius at the acromion is detached widely with a bone block. Next the deltoid muscle is split and the acromion is osteotomized at its midlateral point along the axis of the spine of the scapula. The subacromial space is thus well visualized. The shoulder is elevated to 90 degrees in the scapular plane and a small bony groove is made in the tuberosity. The trapezius is then passed beneath the osteotomized acromion and the supraspinatus, infraspinatus, and subscapularis are sutured to the trapezius flap as needed (**Fig. 5–11**).

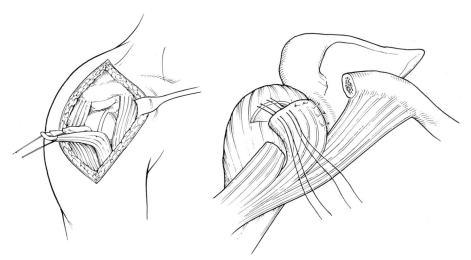

Figure 5–10 Deltoid transfer. The transferred muscle unit is sewn to the residual medial cuff and to the leading edge of the remnant posterior cuff. To ensure a strong construct, the deep fascia of the deltoid must be incorporated into the repair.

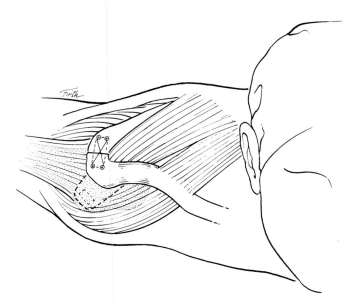

Figure 5–11 Trapezius transfer. The trapezius is harvested from the lateral clavicle and the scapular spine with a small bone block. The subacromial space is accessed via an acromial osteotomy, which is repaired with a tension band technique.

The acromial osteotomy is then fixed with a tension band technique. Passive elevation and rotation are begun on the fifth postoperative day with active exercises started at 4 weeks.[59]

Mikasa and Yamanaka performed seven trapezius transfers for massive RC tears. Their primary indication for transfer was pain at rest and night pain in patients where primary RC repair could not be performed. Preoperatively patients were limited to 77 degrees of flexion and 43 degrees of ER. At an average of 45 months, pain at rest was eliminated in all patients; however, night pain and pain with motion remained in one patient. Average flexion increased to 109 degrees and ER to 60 degrees.[17,60]

Trapezius transfer is a salvage operation with the potential to relieve a patient's pain when the RC tendons cannot be primarily repaired. The trapezius is a synergist of the deltoid muscle and its fibers contract in a similar line of pull as the supraspinatus. Mikasa and Yamanaka found that results improved if the long head of the biceps was preserved. This transfer requires a stable pulley effect only achieved with a healed acromial osteotomy. If the osteotomy does not heal, the trapezius transfer will become a head elevator like the deltoid and the nonunion site may be symptomatic. Additionally, if the patient develops a cuff-tear arthropathy or if the transfer fails, glenohumeral arthrodesis is compromised, and, as a prime contributor to scapulothoracic motion, the trapezius, is lost.

Conclusion

Tendon transfers for irreparable RC tears serve to optimize function and minimize pain. No single transfer has gained wide acceptance, as none offers a perfect solution to the complex dilemma of massive, irreparable, RC tear. Furthermore, there is a paucity of data comparing the various techniques. Individual patient characteristics and the skills and preferences unique to each surgeon should be considered when choosing the most appropriate tendon transfer for irreparable RC tears.

References

1. Paavolainen P. Teres minor transfer. In: Burkhead WZ Jr., ed. Rotator Cuff Disorders. Baltimore, MD: Williams & Wilkins, 1996:342–348
2. Burkhart SS. Arthroscopic treatment of massive rotator cuff tears. Clinical results and biomechanical rationale. Clin Orthop Relat Res 1991;267:45–56
3. Cofield RH. Subscapular muscle transposition for repair of chronic rotator cuff tears. Surg Gynecol Obstet 1982;154(5):667–672
4. Gerber C, Fuchs B, Hodler J. The results of repair of massive tears of the rotator cuff. J Bone Joint Surg Am 2000;82(4):505–515
5. Patte D. Classification of rotator cuff lesions. Clin Orthop Relat Res 1990; 254:81–86
6. Warner JJ. Management of massive irreparable rotator cuff tears: the role of tendon transfer. Instr Course Lect 2001;50:63–71
7. Worland RL, Arredondo J, Angles F, Lopez-Jimenez F. Repair of massive rotator cuff tears in patients older than 70 years. J Shoulder Elbow Surg 1999;8(1):26–30
8. Bigliani LU, Cordasco FA, McIlveen SJ, Musso ES. Operative treatment of failed repairs of the rotator cuff. J Bone Joint Surg Am 1992;74(10):1505–1515
9. Aldridge JM, Atkinson TS, Mallon WJ. Combined pectoralis major and latissimus dorsi tendon transfer for massive rotator cuff deficiency. J Shoulder Elbow Surg 2004;13(6):621–629
10. Handelberg FW. Treatment options in full thickness rotator cuff tears. Acta Orthop Belg 2001;67(2):110–115
11. Burkhart SS. Nottage, W. M.; Ogilvie-Harris, D. J.; Kohn, H. S.; and Pachelli, A.: Partial repair of irreparable rotator cuff tears. Arthroscopy 1994;10(4):363–370
12. Rockwood CA Jr, Williams GR Jr, Burkhead WZ Jr. Debridement of degenerative, irreparable lesions of the rotator cuff. J Bone Joint Surg Am 1995;77(6):857–866
13. Bush LF. The torn shoulder capsule. J Bone Joint Surg Am 1975; 57(2):256–259
14. Debeyre J, Patie D, Elmelik E. Repair of Ruptures of the Rotator Cuff of the Shoulder. J Bone Joint Surg Br 1965;47:36–42
15. Gerber C. Latissimus dorsi transfer for the treatment of irreparable tears of the rotator cuff. Clin Orthop Relat Res 1992; 275:152–160
16. Karas SE. Subscapularis transfer for management of massive rotator cuff tears. In: Burkhead WZ Jr., ed. Rotator Cuff Disorders. Baltimore, MD: Williams & Wilkins; 1996:335–341
17. Mikasa M, Bayley I and Kessel L. Trapezius transfer for global tear of the rotator cuff. In: Bateman JE and Welsh RP, Surgery of the Shoulder. Philadelphia, PA: Decker Ink; 1984: 196–199
18. Celli A, Marongiu MC, Rovesta C, Celli L. Transplant of the teres major in the treatment of irreparable injuries of the rotator cuff

(long-term analysis of results). Chir Organi Mov 2005;90(2):121–132

19. Wirth MA, Rockwood CA Jr. Operative treatment of irreparable rupture of the subscapularis. J Bone Joint Surg Am 1997;79(5):722–731

20. Neviaser RJ, Neviaser TJ. Transfer of the subscapularis and teres minor for massive defects of the rotator cuff. In: Bayley I and Kessel L, Shoulder Surgery. New York, NY: Springer; 1982:681–684

21. Gazielly DF. Deltoid muscular flap transfer for massive defects of the rotator cuff. In: Burkhead WZ Jr., ed. Rotator Cuff Disorders. Baltimore, MD: Williams & Wilkins,1996:356–367

22. Spahn G, Kirschbaum S, Klinger HM. A study for evaluating the effect of the deltoid-flap repair in massive rotator cuff defects. Knee Surg Sports Traumatol Arthrosc 2006;14(4):365–372

23. Walch G, Boulahia A, Calderone S, Robinson AHN. The dropping and hornblower's signs in evaluation of rotator cuff tears. J Bone Joint Surg Br 1988;80(4):624–628

24. Karas SE, Giachello TL. Subscapularis transfer for reconstruction of massive tears of the rotator cuff. J Bone Joint Surg Am 1996;78(2):239–245

25. Neer CS. Impingement lesions. Clin Orthop Relat Res 1983; 173:70–77

26. Edwards TB, Baghian S, Faust DC, Willis RB. Results of latissimus dorsi and teres major transfer to the rotator cuff in the treatment of Erb's palsy. J Pediatr Orthop 2000;20(3):375–379

27. Saha AK. Surgery of the paralysed and flail shoulder. Acta Orthop Scand Suppl 1967;97:5–90

28. Zachary RB. Transplantation of teres major and latissimus dorsi for loss of external rotation at the shoulder. Lancet 1947;2:757–758

29. Gilbert A, Romana C, Ayatti R. Tendon transfers for shoulder paralysis in children. Hand Clin 1988;4(4):633–642

30. Gerber C, Maquieira G, Espinosa N. Latissimus dorsi transfer for the treatment of irreparable rotator cuff tears. J Bone Joint Surg Am 2006;88(1):113–120

31. Bartlett SP, May JW Jr, Yaremchuk MJ. The latissimus dorsi muscle: a fresh cadaver study of the primary neuromuscular pedicle. Plast Reconstr Surg 1981;67:631–636

32. Aoki M, Okamura K, Fukushima S, Takahashi T, Ogino T. Transfer of latissimus dorsi for irreparable rotator-cuff tears. J Bone Joint Surg Br 1996;78(5):761–766

33. Miniaci A, MacLeod M. Transfer of the latissimus dorsi muscle after failed repair of a massive tear of the rotator cuff. A two to five-year review. J Bone Joint Surg Am 1999;81(8):1120–1127

34. Warner JJ, Parsons IM. Latissimus dorsi tendon transfer: a comparative analysis of primary and salvage reconstruction of massive, irreparable rotator cuff tears. J Shoulder Elbow Surg 2001;10(6):514–521

35. Codman EA. The Shoulder. 2nd ed. Boston, MA: Thomas Todd Co.; 1934:262–312

36. Frankle MA, Cofield RH. Rotator cuff tears including the subscapularis. In: Proceedings of the Fifth International Conference on Surgery of the Shoulder. Paris, France: International Shoulder and Elbow Society, 1992;52

37. Deutsch A, Altchek DW, Veltri DM, Potter HG, Warren RF. Traumatic tears of the subscapularis tendon. Clinical diagnosis, magnetic resonance imaging findings, and operative treatment. Am J Sports Med 1997;25(1):13–22

38. Gerber C, Hersche O, Farron A. Isolated rupture of the subscapularis tendon. J Bone Joint Surg Am 1996;78(7):1015–1023

39. Burkhart SS. Fluoroscopic comparison of kinematic patterns in massive rotator cuff tears. A suspension bridge model. Clin Orthop Relat Res 1992; 284:144–152

40. Jost B, Puskas GJ, Lustenberger A, Gerber C. Outcome of pectoralis major transfer for the treatment of irreparable subscapularis tears. J Bone Joint Surg Am 2003;85-A(10):1944–1951

41. Resch H, Povacz P, Ritter E, Matschi W. Transfer of the pectoralis major muscle for the treatment of irreparable rupture of the subscapularis tendon. J Bone Joint Surg Am 2000;82(3):372–382

42. Hoffman GW, Elliott LF. The anatomy of the pectoral nerves and its significance to the general and plastic surgeon. Ann Surg 1987;205(5):504–507

43. Gerber C, Vinh TS, Hertel R, and Hess CW. Latissimus dorsi transfer for the treatment of massive tears of the rotator cuff. A preliminary report. Clin Orthop Relat Res 1988, 232:51–61

44. L'Episcopo JB. Tendon transplantation in obstetrical paralysis. Am J Surg 1934;25:122–125

45. Hartrampf CR, Elliott LF, Feldman S. A triceps musculocutaneous flap for chest-wall defects. Plast Reconstr Surg 1990;86(3):502–509

46. Miller DV. Discussion: The use of the long head of the triceps interposition muscle flap for treatment of massive rotator cuff tears. Plast Reconstr Surg 1990;110:1120–1127

47. Malkani AL, Sundine MJ, Tillett ED, Baker DL, Rogers RA, Morton A. Transfer of the long head of the triceps tendon for irreparable rotator cuff tears. Clin Orthop Relat Res 2004; 428: 228–236

48. Travill AA. Electromyographic study of the extensor apparatus of the forearm. Anat Rec 1962;144:373–376

49. Keating JF, Waterworth P, Shaw-Dunn J, Crossan J. The relative strengths of the rotator cuff muscles. A cadaver study. J Bone Joint Surg Br 1993;75(1):137–140

50. Ha'eri GB, Wiley AM. Advancement of the supraspinatus muscle in the repair of ruptures of the rotator cuff. J Bone Joint Surg Am 1981;63(2):232–238

51. Otis JC, Jiang CC, Wickiewicz TL, Peterson MG, Warren RF, Santner TJ. Changes in the moment arms of the rotator cuff and deltoid muscles with abduction and rotation. J Bone Joint Surg Am 1994;76(5):667–676

52. Hansen PE. Biceps transfer interposition grafting in massive rotator cuff tears. In: Burkhead WZ Jr., Rotator Cuff Disorders. Baltimore, MD: Williams & Wilkins: 1996:342–348

53. Ellman H, Hanker G, Bayer M. Repair of the rotator cuff. J Bone Joint Surg Am 1985;67:974–979

54. Kumar VP, Satku K, Balasubramaniam P. The role of the long head of biceps brachii in the stabilization of the head of the humerus. Clin Orthop Relat Res 1989; 244:172–175

55. Augereau B. Traitement Chirurgical des Ruptures de la Coiffe des Rotateurs. Cahiers d'Enseignement SOFCOT. Paris, France: Expansion Scientifique Francaise 1989 (Abstract 161): 161

56. Takagishi N. The new operation for the massive rotator cuff rupture. J Jap Orthop Assoc. 1978;52:775–780

57. Saragaglia D, Tourne Y. Transfer of the deltoid muscular flap for massive defects of the rotator cuff: 27 patients. In: Fifth International Conference on Surgery of the Shoulder. Paris, France: July 12–15, 1993

58. Mansat P, Frankle MA, Cofield RH. Tears in the subscapularis tendon: descriptive analysis and results of surgical repair. Joint Bone Spine 2003;70(5):342–347

59. Yamanaka K, Mikasa M. Trapezius transfer. In: Burkhead WZ Jr, Rotator Cuff Disorders. Baltimore, MD: Williams & Wilkins, 1996: 374–379

60. Mikasa M. Trapezius transfer for global tear of the rotator cuff. In: Bateman JE and Welsh RP, Surgery of the Shoulder. Philadelphia, PA: BC Decker, 1984:196–199

61. Bjorkenheim JM, Paavolainen P, Ahovuo J, Slatis P. Surgical repair of the rotator cuff and surrounding tissues. Factors influencing the results. Clin Orthop Relat Res 1988; 236:148–153

62. Galatz LM, Ball CM, Teefey SA, Middleton WD, Yamaguchi K. The outcome and repair integrity of completely arthroscopically repaired large and massive rotator cuff tears. J Bone Joint Surg Am 2004;86-A(2):219–224

63. Gartsman GM, Khan M, Hammerman SM. Arthroscopic repair of full-thickness tears of the rotator cuff. J Bone Joint Surg Am 2000;82:304–314

64. Harryman DT, Mack LA, Wang KY, Jackins SE, Richardson ML, Matsen FA. Repairs of the rotator cuff. Correlation of functional results with integrity of the cuff. J Bone Joint Surg Am 1991;73(7):982–989

65. Rokito AS, Cuomo F, Gallagher MA, Zuckerman JD. Long-term functional outcome of repair of large and massive chronic tears of the rotator cuff. J Bone Joint Surg Am 1999;81(7):991–997

66. Tauro JC. Arthroscopic rotator cuff repair: analysis of technique and results at 2- and 3-year follow-up. Arthroscopy 1998;14:45–51

67. Liu J, Hughes RE, O'Driscoll SW, An KN. Biomechanical effect of medial advancement of the supraspinatus tendon. A study in cadavera. J Bone Joint Surg Am 1998;80(6):853–859

68. Gerber C, Hersche O. Tendon transfers for the treatment of irreparable rotator cuff defects. Orthop Clin North Am 1997;28(2):195–203

69. Mikasa M. Long-term results of surgical treatment for massive rotator cuff tears. With special reference to trapezius transfers. Clin Orthop Surg 1989;24:38–45

70. Mikasa M. Experience of the trapezius transfer for the massive rotator cuff tear. The Shoulder Joint 1979; 3:77–80

71. Magermans DJ, Chadwick EK, Veeger HE, Rozing PM, Van der Helm FC. Effectiveness of tendon transfers for massive rotator cuff tears: a simulation study. Clin Biomech (Bristol, Avon) 2004;19(2):116–122

72. Wang AA, Strauch RJ, Flatow EL, Bigliani LU, Rosenwasser MP. The teres major muscle: an anatomic study of its use as a tendon transfer. J Shoulder Elbow Surg 1999;8:334–338

73. Pagnotta A, Haerle M, Gilbert A. Long-term results on abduction and external rotation of the shoulder after latissimus dorsi transfer for sequelae of obstetric palsy. Clin Orthop Relat Res 2004; 426:199–205

74. Waters PM, Bae DS. Effect of tendon transfers and extra-articular soft-tissue balancing on glenohumeral development in brachial plexus birth palsy. J Bone Joint Surg Am 2005;87(2):320–325

75. Cleeman E, Hazrati Y, Auerbach JD, Shubin SK, Hausman M, Flatow EL. Latissimus dorsi tendon transfer for massive rotator cuff tears: a cadaveric study. J Shoulder Elbow Surg 2003;12(6):539–543

76. Pearle AD, Kelly BT, Voos JE, Chehab EL, Warren RF. Surgical technique and anatomic study of latissimus dorsi and teres major transfers. J Bone Joint Surg Am 2006;88(7):1524–1531

77. Rowsell AR, Eisenberg N, Davies DM, Taylor GI. The anatomy of the thoracodorsal artery within the latissimus dorsi muscle. Br J Plast Surg 1986;39:206–209

78. Tobin GR, Schusterman M, Peterson GH, Nichols G, Bland KI. The intramuscular neurovascular anatomy of the latissimus dorsi muscle: the basis for splitting the flap. Plast Reconstr Surg 1981;67:637–641

79. Gerber C, Krushell RJ. Isolated rupture of the tendon of the subscapularis muscle. Clinical features in 16 cases. J Bone Joint Surg Br 1991;73(3):389–394

6

The Spectrum of Disease in the Rotator Cuff–Deficient Shoulder

Jonathan Levy

The understanding of the relationship between the rotator cuff (RC) deficient shoulder and glenohumeral arthritis continues to evolve. Early attempts at defining this pathology resulted in a variety of nomenclature used to describe a similar clinical presentation: Milwaukee shoulder, l'épaule sénile hémorragique (the hemorrhagic shoulder of the elderly), cuff tear arthropathy (CTA), apatite-associated destructive arthritis, and so on. These clinical descriptions were focused on disease characteristics that typify what has become known as CTA: severe glenohumeral arthritis with joint collapse, a hemorrhagic-crystalline effusion, and a massive RC tear. Classic CTA actually represents one of several disease processes that can be present in the rotator cuff deficient shoulder. In fact, a spectrum of disease exists for the RC-deficient shoulder (**Fig. 6–1**).

Classic CTA, as originally described by Neer and colleagues,[1] represents the patient with a massive RC tear with severe glenohumeral arthritis that advances with collapse of the articular surface. However, several other manifestations within the spectrum of the RC-deficient shoulder may result in a similar loss of function (**Table 6–1**). These include instability due to massive RC tears, RC tears with minimal arthritis, RC deficiency with anterior superior escape, and a variety of conditions that result in proximal humeral bone loss and subsequent RC deficiency (i.e., nonunion of greater tuberosity or tumor resection).

My goal in this chapter is to first review the established knowledge on the disease. I will then focus on utilizing my group's experience in managing this population of patients to establish key principles necessary to understand the pathology, pathophysiology, and treatment of the RC-deficient shoulder. By clearly defining the pathology present, one can begin to understand how aspects of the pathology contribute to the pathophysiology of the disease. This introduction will serve as a foundation for other chapters, as these principals are paramount in the diagnosis and management of the RC-deficient shoulder.

Historical Background

Although Neer et al[1] first coined the term *cuff tear arthropathy*, the description of such pathology was reported previously. In the 19th century, Adams and Smith described a patient with a localized form of rheumatoid arthritis involving the shoulder.[2–5] In 1934, Codman reported a patient with a subacromial space hygroma who had recurrent swelling, RC deficiency, severe glenohumeral arthritis, and cartilaginous bodies of the synovium.[3] In 1981, McCarty coined the term *Milwaukee shoulder* seen in 4 patients with identical clinical presentations and joint fluid with active collagenase, neutral proteinase, and hydroxyapatite crystals.[4] In 1983, Neer et al[1] introduced the term *cuff tear arthropathy* to describe the presentation of 26 patients with massive RC tears and glenohumeral arthritis treated with a total shoulder replacement. Over the last century, several reports of similar clinical presentations established various theories as to how patients developed the condition.

Classic Cuff Tear Arthropathy

Several theories on the etiology of CTA have been discussed. There exists no consensus among reports. The rheumatologic literature has emphasized the biochemical aspects of the condition, whereas the orthopedic descriptions have emphasized the mechanical factors.[5–12]

Reports of a hemorrhagic theory for CTA focused on the presence of a hemarthrosis in patients with severe glenohumeral arthritis and massive RC tears. In 1967, DeSeze[6] first described this in 3 patients; however, later reports by Baudin[5] in 1969 and Lamboley[7] in 1977 noted similar presentations.

Another group of reports focused on the inflammatory nature of the disease process. The Milwaukee shoulder was introduced in the rheumatology literature by McCarty in 1981.[4] This condition, reported mostly in women, consisted of massive RC tear, glenohumeral arthritis, bony destruction, and joint instability. The hemarthrosis present contained calcium phosphate crystals, active collagenase, protease activity, and inflammatory cells.[4,8,9] The description of the Milwaukee shoulder emphasized the central role of calcium phosphate crystals. These crystals are phagocytized by synovial cells activating the release of destructive enzymes, which act on periarticular tissue and joint surfaces.[4,8–17] Antoniou et al[10] noted an association between the apatite crystals, massive RC tears, and glenohumeral arthritis. These crystals were seen with high levels of PGE2 in the synovial fluid of patients with CTA. The result is a picture of severe degenerative arthritis with significant bone loss and soft tissue destruction.

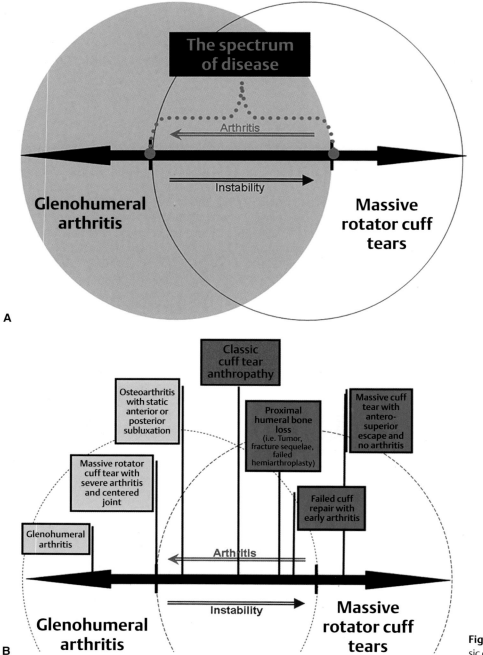

Figure 6–1 (A) The spectrum of disease. **(B)** Classic cuff tear arthroplasty.

The nutritional theory emphasizes the role of the RC as a structural barrier. As noted by Neer and colleagues,[1] extravasation of synovial fluid in the presence of massive RC tears results in an inadequate diffusion of nutritional components necessary for articular cartilage metabolism. Additionally, by not using the joint, alterations in articular content (i.e., water content) and disuse osteopenia develop. This results in cartilage atrophy, subchondral osteopenia, and collapse of the humeral head.

Perhaps the most significant role that the RC plays in CTA is described in the mechanical theory. Neer et al[1] was the first to emphasize this role. The instability that results from RC deficiency is the first step toward the development of CTA. Loss of RC function results in a loss of the balanced force couples needed to establish a stable fulcrum for the glenohumeral joint.[11] In this setting, the deltoid moment results in glenohumeral instability with excessive upward migration of the humeral head. Mechanical factors of glenohumeral instability from RC dysfunction and proximal migration of the humeral head to the point of acromial impingement result in degenerative changes seen on the humeral head, superior glenoid, and undersur-

Table 6–1   Other Presentations of Cuff Deficient Shoulder

Tendon loss

Massive rotator cuff tear with minimal arthritis

Massive rotator cuff tear with anterosuperior escape

Infection

Muscle loss

Infection

Severe glenohumeral arthritis with severe fatty infiltration of intact rotator cuff

Bone loss

Fracture sequelae

Failed hemiarthroplasty for fracture

Failed hemiarthroplasty with rotator cuff tear

Failed hemiarthroplasty for cuff tear arthropathy

Failed bipolar hemiarthroplasty

Tumor resection

Infection

Nerve loss

Chronic Erb palsy

Suprascapular nerve palsy

Post-polio

face of the acromion. The end result is acetabularization of the shoulder joint with severe joint destruction.

The connection between massive RC tears and the development of classic CTA has not been clearly elucidated. Neer et al[1] estimated that 4% of patients with RC tears would develop CTA. Hamada and colleagues,[12] however, noted progressive degenerative changes in 5 of 7 patients with massive RC tears, suggesting that massive RC tears would ultimately lead to progressive degenerative changes. In a cadaveric study, Feeney et al[13] showed a strong correlation between tears of the RC and articular cartilage degenerative changes, as they found articular cartilage damage in all 10 shoulders that had RC tears. Nonetheless, Rockwood and colleagues[14] noted no progression of glenohumeral degeneration in patients with massive RC tears 6.5 years after open acromioplasty and débridement of the RC. The mere presence of a massive RC tear may not be enough to develop the progressive degenerative changes seen in classic CTA; however, these massive tears may result in severe functional loss. One would suspect that as the aging population increases, the incidence of problems related to the RC-deficient shoulder will surge.

Other Disease Presentations of the Rotator Cuff Deficient Shoulder

Several conditions result in disability due to RC deficiency (**Table 6–1**). The central role of the RC in providing shoul-

der function is clear. RC deficiency results in variable degrees of weakness and instability that result in a significant loss of function for the patient. Burkhart introduced the concept of balanced force couples to distinguish functional from dysfunctional massive RC tears.[15] Once a balanced force couple is lost, the RC becomes dysfunctional.

Whether the massive RC tear occurs with minimal arthritis, severe arthritis (i.e., classic CTA), or isolated instability (i.e., anterosuperior escape), the function of the RC will ultimately determine the functional outcome. Reconstructive options must strongly consider the ability to restore a functional RC for reliable improvements to be achieved.

In cases where the RC tendon is intact, severe muscular atrophy of the RC may result in its dysfunction. This has been recognized in patients with severe osteoarthritis and an intact RC.[16,17] In these patients when the arthritis is treated with a total shoulder arthroplasty, instability results. It is thought that the friction created by the severe arthritis creates a static stability. When this friction is replaced with a smooth articulating surface, RC dysfunction results in joint instability and failure of the joint replacement.

RC deficiency may also develop after failure of a RC repair or subacromial decompression. This may be the result of the natural history of the disease. However, the important role of the coracoacromial arch in preventing anterosuperior instability of the glenohumeral joint has been described.[18] In cases where both the RC and the coracoacromial arch are deficient, the resulting anterosuperior instability results in significant disability and loss of shoulder function, often with pseudoparesis of the shoulder.

Several disease processes result in significant proximal humeral bone loss. The importance of proximal humeral bone is based on the RC insertion. As proximal humeral bone loss becomes more severe, the loss of RC insertion becomes greater. In severe cases of proximal humeral bone loss, significant weakness and instability will result. This is seen in cases of proximal humeral tuberosity malunion, nonunion, or resorption, where the RC becomes dysfunctional due to loss of its secure attachment. Similar findings are seen in cases of failed hemiarthroplasty for proximal humerus fracture, after tumor resection, and as a result of infection. Infections of the shoulder can be particularly devastating, as loss of RC is coupled with significant joint destruction and bone loss with limited reconstructive options.

Classification of Rotator Cuff Deficiency

To date, the only attempts at classifying RC deficiency have been based on radiographic classifications. Two attempts have been made to classify the RC-deficient shoulder into distinct radiographic groups.[19,20] It has been reported that these radiographic distinctions may help to guide shoulder surgeons in selection of appropriate treatment plan.[20] Both radiographic classification systems describe several grades of degeneration, bone loss, and fixed instability.

In 1990, Hameda et al[19] proposed the first classification of massive RC tears. The classification was based on a series of 22 massive cuff tears that were treated nonoperatively. Five radiographic grades were described (**Fig. 6–2**). They noted progression to CTA in one patient. They concluded that patients with massive RC tears will ultimately progress to CTA. Along the way, progressive radiographic changes develop due to rupture of the long head of the biceps, establishment of an abnormal fulcrum of the humeral head against the acromion and the coracoacromial ligament, and progressive weakness of external rotation.[19]

Seebauer et al[20] was the first to emphasize the importance of joint stability. The Seebauer classification of CTA (**Fig. 6–3**) has four radiographic stages with two types and two subtypes. Patients with type 1 have centered joints that are stable, whereas patients with type II have lost stability of the joint. Patients with type IA have developed acetabularization of the coracoacromial arch with rounding of the humeral head. These patients have maintained joint stability with intact anterior structures as noted by the minimal amounts of superior migration of the humeral head. Type IB differs in progressive loss of the anterior restraints. These patients have compromised, but main-

tained dynamic joint stabilization with minimal superior migration of the humeral head. As the anterior structures of the shoulder become compromised, progressive instability results. Thus patients with type IIA and type IIB show radiographic evidence of fixed instability. In type IIA, superomedial erosion and extensive acetabularization of the coracoacromial arch are seen. The humeral head is superior translated. Instability is the hallmark of type IIB, as the arthritic changes are minimal. The humeral head is described in an anterosuperior position due to a deficient coracoacromial arch.[20]

The Seebauer classification has been used to establish algorithms for the management of CTA.[20,21] Based on these algorithms, patients with type IA can be successfully managed using hemiarthroplasty, because the joint remains centered. On the other hand, patients with radiographs classified as type IIB should be managed with a reverse prosthesis to treat the underlying joint instability.

The use of any radiographic classification system as a treatment algorithm should be done so with caution. Treatment of CTA requires a clear understanding of the pathology present. Although aspects of this are seen on radiographs (i.e., bone loss and loss of smooth articulat-

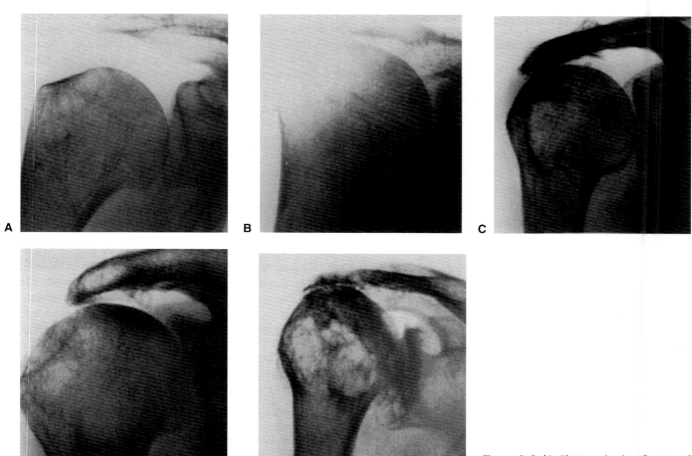

A

B

C

D

E

Figure 6–2 (A–E) Hamada classification of massive rotator cuff tears.

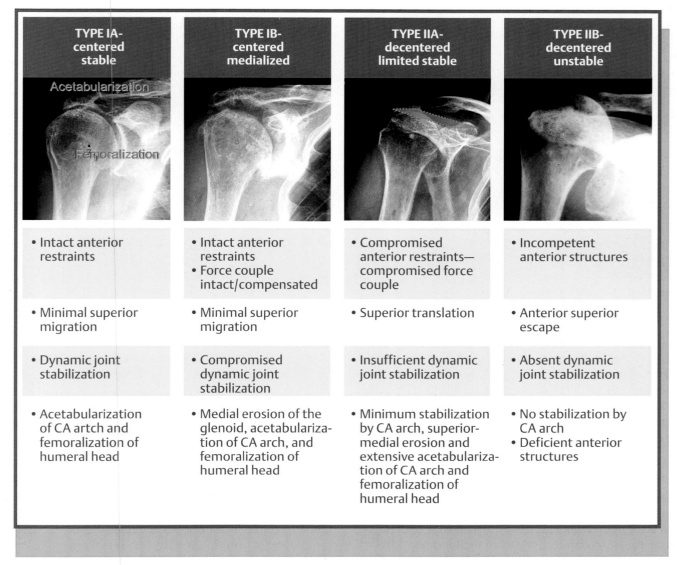

TYPE IA- centered stable	TYPE IB- centered medialized	TYPE IIA- decentered limited stable	TYPE IIB- decentered unstable
• Intact anterior restraints	• Intact anterior restraints • Force couple intact/compensated	• Compromised anterior restraints— compromised force couple	• Incompetent anterior structures
• Minimal superior migration	• Minimal superior migration	• Superior translation	• Anterior superior escape
• Dynamic joint stabilization	• Compromised dynamic joint stabilization	• Insufficient dynamic joint stabilization	• Absent dynamic joint stabilization
• Acetabularization of CA artch and femoralization of humeral head	• Medial erosion of the glenoid, acetabulariza- tion of CA arch, and femoralization of humeral head	• Minimum stabilization by CA arch, superior- medial erosion and extensive acetabulariza- tion of CA arch and femoralization of humeral head	• No stabilization by CA arch • Deficient anterior structures

Figure 6–3 Seebauer classification of cuff tear arthropathy. CA, coracoacromial. From Visotsky JL, Basamania C, Seebauer L, Rockwood CA Jr., Jensen KL. Cuff tear arthropathy: pathogenesis, classification, and algorithm for treatment. J Bone Joint Surg Am 2004; 86:38. Adapted by permission.

ing surfaces), much of the pathology is not seen. A clear example is a patient with anterosuperior instability due to RC and coracoacromial arch deficiency. This patient may have seemingly normal radiographs (**Fig. 6–4**). This radiograph does not fit into any current classification system. However, when a dynamic radiograph is performed in attempted forward elevation, the dynamic instability clearly becomes evident (**Fig. 6–5**).

Although radiographic classification systems may be useful, they do not accurately represent the spectrum of disease seen in the RC-deficient shoulder. To classify RC deficiency accurately, a proper understanding of the pathology present is necessary. A more reliable classifica-

tion system would grade each of the pathological changes present and incorporate relevant radiographic findings.

Pathology

Identification and understanding the pathological changes seen in the RC-deficient shoulder are essential for proper diagnosis and management of the disease. The structures that may undergo pathological change include the RC muscle and tendon, articular surfaces of the glenohumeral joint, bone support of the glenoid and humeral head, surrounding capsule, position of the glenohumeral joint, the deltoid

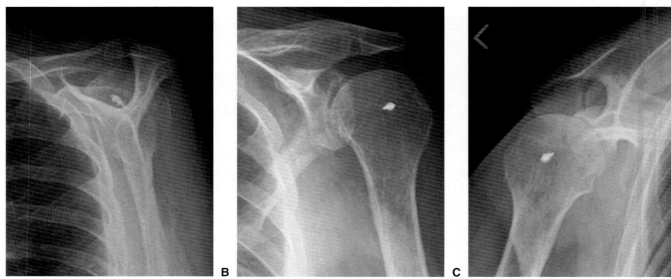

Figure 6–4 Static anteroposterior **(A)**, Y **(B)**, and axillary **(C)** radiographs of 6-month follow-up after subacromial decompression and mini-open rotator cuff repair.

muscle, and the subdeltoid, subacromial, and subcoracoid space (**Table 6–2**). Each of these pathological changes plays significant roles in the disease process and may dramatically influence selection of treatment plan. Once the extent of the pathology present in the involved shoulder can be asserted, information from the clinical picture can be integrated to form a logical treatment strategy.

Loss of Rotator Cuff Muscle and Tendon

The essential component of RC deficiency is directly related to the amount of RC function lost. The size of the RC tendon tear is the most obvious aspect of this pathology, because the larger the RC tendon tear, the more the functional loss.[22,23] However, the degree of muscle loss may be even more signifi-

cant. Fatty infiltration of the RC muscle after RC tendon tears has been previously described by Goutallier et al[24] based on computed tomography (CT) scans (**Table 6–3**). These muscular changes seen after RC tendon tears may be irreversible, even after a successful tendon repair.[25,26] A critical level of RC muscle and tendon loss will result in significant functional loss including weakness and joint instability.[27]

In patients with RC deficiency, the RC is unable to provide these important roles. Reconstructive efforts must thus consider whether these functions can be reliably restored, or whether efforts should be made to compensate for the loss of strength and stability. Once instability has developed from RC deficiency, the reliability of soft tissue procedures at restoring stability becomes diminished. Preoperative magnetic resonance imaging (MRI) or CT scans

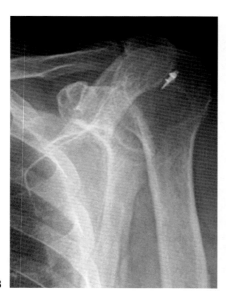
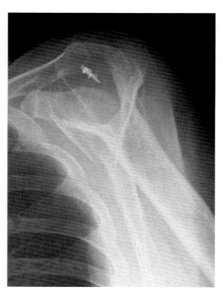

Figure 6–5 Dynamic forward elevation anteroposterior **(A)** and Y **(B)** radiographs demonstrating clear anterosuperior escape.

38. Pollock RG, Deliz ED, McIlveen SJ, Flatow EL, Bigliani LU. Prosthetic replacement in rotator cuff-deficient shoulders. J Shoulder Elbow Surg 1992;1:173–186

39. Sanchez-Sotelo J, Cofield RH, Rowland CM. Shoulder hemiarthroplasty for glenohumeral arthritis associated with severe rotator cuff deficiency. J Bone Joint Surg Am 2001;83-A(12):1814–1822

40. Caporali R, Rossi S, Montecucco C. Tidal irrigation in Milwaukee shoulder syndrome. J Rheumatol 1994;21(9):1781–1782

41. Ellman H, Kay SP, Wirth M. Arthroscopic treatment of full-thickness rotator cuff tears: 2- to 7-year follow-up study. Arthroscopy 1993;9:195–200

42. Melillo AS, Savoie FH, Field LD. Massive rotator cuff tears: debridement versus repair. Orthop Clin North Am 1997;28:117–124

43. Zvijac JE, Levy HJ, Lemak LJ. Arthroscopic subacromial decompression in the treatment of full thickness rotator cuff tears: a 3- to 6-year follow-up. Arthroscopy 1994;10(5):518–523

44. Walch G, Edwards TB, Boulahia A, Nove-Josserand L, Neyton L, Szabo I. Arthroscopic tenotomy of the long head of the biceps in the treatment of rotator cuff tears: clinical and radiographic results of 307 cases. J Shoulder Elbow Surg 2005;14(3):238–246

45. Scheibe IM, Lichtenberg S, Habermeyer P. Reversed arthroscopic subacromial decompression for massive rotator cuff tears. J Shoulder Elbow Surg 2004;13(3):272–278

46. Fenlin JM, Chase JM, Rushton SA, Frieman BG. Tuberoplasty: creation of an acromiohumeral articulation—a treatment option for massive, irreparable rotator cuff tears. J Shoulder Elbow Surg 2002;11:136–142

47. Burkhart SS, Nottage WM, Ogilvie-Harris DJ, Kohn HS, Pachelli A. Partial repair of irreparable rotator cuff tears. Arthroscopy 1994;10(4):363–370

48. Rockwood CA, Lyons FR. Shoulder impingement syndrome: diagnosis, radiographic evaluation and treatment with a modified Neer acromioplasty. J Bone Joint Surg Am 1993;75:409–424

49. Gartsman GM. Massive, irreparable tears of the rotator cuff. Results of operative débridement and subacromial decompression. J Bone Joint Surg Am 1997;79:715–721

50. Neviaser JS, Neviaser RJ, Neviaser TJ. The repair of chronic massive ruptures of the rotator cuff of the shoulder by use of freeze-dried rotator cuff. J Bone Joint Surg Am 1978;60-A:681–684

51. Gerber C, Maquieira G, Espinosa N. Latissimus dorsi transfer for the treatment of irreparable rotator cuff tears. J Bone Joint Surg Am 2006;88(1):113–120

52. Warner JP. Management of massive irreparable rotator cuff tears: the role of tendon transfer. J Bone Joint Surg Am 2000;82(6):878–887

53. Jost B, Puskas GJ, Lustenberger A, Gerber C. Outcome of pectoralis major transfer for the treatment of irreparable subscapularis tears. J Bone Joint Surg Am 2003;85-A(10):1944–1951

54. Galatz LM, Connor PM, Calfee RP, Hsu JC, Yamaguchi K. Pectoralis major transfer for anterior-superior subluxation in massive rotator cuff insufficiency. J Shoulder Elbow Surg 2003;12(1):1–5

55. Arntz CT, Matsen FA III, Jackins S. Surgical management of complex irreparable rotator cuff deficiency. J Arthroplasty 1991;6:363–370

56. Cofield RH, Briggs BT. Glenohumeral arthrodesis: operative and long-term functional results. J Bone Joint Surg Am 1979;61:668–677

57. Richards RR, Waddell JP, Hudson AR. Shoulder arthrodesis for the treatment of brachial plexus palsy. Clin Orthop Relat Res 1985;198:250–258

58. Barrett WP, Franklin JL, Jackins SE, Wyss CR, Matsen FA III. Total shoulder arthroplasty. J Bone Joint Surg Am 1987;69:865–872

59. Franklin JL, Barrett WP, Jackins SE, Matsen FA III. Glenoid loosening in total shoulder arthroplasty. Association with rotator cuff deficiency. J Arthroplasty 1988;3:39–46

60. Arntz CT, Jackins S, Matsen FA III. Prosthetic replacement of the shoulder for the treatment of defects in the rotator cuff and the surface of the glenohumeral joint. J Bone Joint Surg Am 1993;75:485–491

61. Field LD, Dines DM, Zabinski SJ, Warren RF. Hemiarthroplasty of the shoulder for rotator cuff arthropathy. J Shoulder Elbow Surg 1997;6:18–23

62. Zuckerman JD, Scott AJ, Gallagher MA. Hemiarthroplasty for cuff tear arthropathy. J Shoulder Elbow Surg 2000;9:169–172

63. Sanchez-Sotelo J, Cofield RH, Rowland CM. Shoulder hemiarthroplasty for glenohumeral arthritis associated with severe rotator cuff deficiency. J Bone Joint Surg Am 2001;83-A(12):1814–1822

64. Lee DH, Niemann KM. Bipolar shoulder arthroplasty. Clin Orthop Relat Res 1994;304:97–107

65. Brostrom LA, Wallensten R, Olsson E, Anderson D. The Kessel prosthesis in total shoulder arthroplasty. A five-year experience. Clin Orthop Relat Res 1992;277:155–160

66. Boileau P, Watkinson DJ, Hatzidakis AM, Balg F. Grammont reverse prosthesis: design, rationale, and biomechanics. J Shoulder Elbow Surg 2005;14:147S–161S

67. Adams R. A Treatise of Rheumatic Gout or Chronic Rheumatic Arthritis of All the Joints. 2nd ed. London: John Churchill and Sons; 1873:91–175

68. Smith RW. Observations upon chronic rheumatic arthritis of the shoulder. Part I. Dublin Quart J Med Sci 1853;15:1–16

69. Smith RW. Observations upon chronic rheumatic arthritis of the shoulder. Part II. Dublin Quart J Med Sci 1853;15:343–358

70. Halverson PB, Carrera GF, McCarty DJ. Milwaukee shoulder syndrome. Arch Intern Med 1990;150:665–672

71. Newman JH, Chavin KD, Chavin IF. Milwaukee shoulder syndrome: a new crystal-induced arthritis syndrome associated with hydroxyapatite crystals: a case report. Del Med J 1983;55:167–169

72. Rachow JW, Ryan LM, McCarty DJ, et al. Synovial fluid inorganic pyrophosphate concentration and nucleotide pyrophosphohydrolase activity in basic calcium phosphate deposition arthropathy and Milwaukee shoulder syndrome. Arthritis Rheum 1988;31:408–413

73. Jensen KL, Williams GR, Russel IJ, Rockwood CA. Current concepts review—rotator cuff tear arthropathy. J Bone Joint Surg Am 1999;81:1312–1324

74. Neviaser RJ, Neviaser TJ, Neviaser JS. Anterior dislocation of the shoulder and rotator cuff rupture. Clin Orthop Relat Res 1993;291:103–106

75. Symeonides P. The significance of the subscapularis muscle in the pathogenesis of recurrent anterior dislocation of the shoulder. J Bone Joint Surg 1972;54B:476–482

76. Williams GR Jr, Rockwood CA Jr. Hemiarthroplasty in rotator cuff-deficient shoulders. J Shoulder Elbow Surg 1996;5:362–367

77. Zuckerman JD, Scott AJ, Gallagher MA. Hemiarthroplasty for cuff tear arthropathy. J Shoulder Elbow Surg 2000;9:169–172

78. Ozaki J, Fujimoto S, Masuhara K, Tamia S, Yoshimoto S. Reconstruction of chronic massive rotator cuff tears with synthetic materials. Clin Orthop Relat Res 1986;202:173–183

79. Sclamberg SG, Tibone JE, Itamura JM, Kasraeian S. Six-month magnetic resonance imaging follow-up of large and massive rotator cuff repairs reinforced with porcine small intestinal submucosa. J Shoulder Elbow Surg 2004;13(5):538–541

80. Wick M, Müller EJ, Ambacher T, Hebler U, Muhr G, Kutscha-Lissberg F. Arthrodesis of the shoulder after septic arthritis: long-term results. J Bone Joint Surg Br 2003;85:666–670

81. Diaz JA, Cohen SB, Warren RF, Craig EV, Allen AA. Arthrodesis as a salvage procedure for recurrent instability of the shoulder. J Shoulder Elbow Surg 2003;12:237–241

82. Safran O, Iannotti JP. Arthrodesis of the shoulder. J Am Acad Orthop Surg 2006;14(3):145–153

83. Pollock RG, Deliz ED, McIlveen SJ, Flatow EL, Bigliani LU. Prosthetic replacement in rotator cuff-deficient shoulders. J Shoulder Elbow Surg 1992;1:173–186

84. Williams GR Jr, Rockwood CA Jr. Hemiarthroplasty in rotator cuff-deficient shoulders. J Shoulder Elbow Surg 1996;5:362–367

85. Sarris IK, Papadimitriou NG, Sotereanos DG. Bipolar hemiarthroplasty for chronic rotator cuff tear arthropathy. J Arthroplasty 2003;18:169–173

86. Worland RL, Jessup DE, Arredondo J, Warburton KJ. Bipolar shoulder arthroplasty for rotator cuff arthropathy. J Shoulder Elbow Surg 1997;6:512–515

87. Frankle M, Siegal S, Pupello D, Saleem A, Mighell M, Vasey M. The reverse shoulder prosthesis for glenohumeral arthritis associated with severe rotator cuff deficiency. A minimum two-year follow-up study of sixty patients. J Bone Joint Surg Am 2005;87(8):1697–1705

88. Werner CM, Steinmann PA, Gilbart M, Gerber C. Treatment of painful pseudoparesis due to irreparable rotator cuff dysfunction with the Delta III reverse-ball-and-socket total shoulder prosthesis. J Bone Joint Surg Am 2005;87(7):1476–1486

89. Sirveaux F, Favard L, Oudet D, Huquet D, Walch G, Mole D. Grammont inverted total shoulder arthroplasty in the treatment of glenohumeral osteoarthritis with massive rupture of the cuff. Results of a multicentre study of 80 shoulders. J Bone Joint Surg Br 2004;86(3):388–395

7 Hemiarthroplasty for Rotator Cuff–Tear Arthropathy

Kamal I. Bohsali, Jeffrey L. Visotsky, Carl J. Basamania, Michael A. Wirth, and Charles A. Rockwood Jr.

In 1853, Adams initially described rotator cuff arthropathy (RCA), when he observed individuals with chronic rotator cuff (RC) tears leading to severe arthritis.[1,2] The term *cuff–tear arthropathy*, however, was coined by Neer and colleagues in 1977 and formally described in 1983.[3] Neer et al reported on the pathoanatomical changes that occurred with chronic massive RC tears, including structural changes in the humeral head (atrophic cartilage, osteoporotic subchondral bone), coracoacromial arch, and glenoid (absent cartilage and sclerosis at point of contact with humeral head) surfaces. Superior displacement of the humerus into the subacromial space resulted in erosion of the greater tuberosity (femoralization), and subsequent morphological changes to the coracoacromial arch (acetabularization) (**Fig. 7–1**).[3] Clinical manifestations included shoulder swelling, supraspinatus and infraspinatus atrophy (weak abduction and external rotation [ER]), as well as limited, incongruous glenohumeral motion with debilitating (at times progressive) pain. Based upon their clinical observations and intraoperative examinations while performing 26 arthroplasties, Neer and coauthors estimated that ~4% of patients with massive RC tears would develop this pathological situation if untreated.[3] Neer et al hypothesized that the presence of two interdependent mechanisms, mechanical and nutri-

tional, contributed to the cyclical process of RC destruction and arthropathy. Radiographic (fluoroscopy, arthrography) and electromyographic analyses of RC tears in patients have provided information to support the force couple theory.[4,5] An imbalance in transverse forces between the subscapularis and posteroinferior cuff or coronal forces between the deltoid and supraspinatus would result in displeasing kinematics. Unstable shoulder kinematics would lead to further wear and accelerated disruption of transverse and coronal plane force couples (**Fig. 7–2**).[4,5]

Classification

Because the outcomes from the treatment of massive RC tears with glenohumeral arthritis are highly variable, attempts have been made to categorize the severity of the RCA. Seebauer and colleagues retrospectively analyzed all institutional patients with RCA treated with conventional hemiarthroplasty. Based upon functional outcomes and radiographs, the authors proposed a biomechanical classification of the RC-deficient arthritic shoulder.[6,7] The four subtypes (Ia, Ib, IIa, IIb) were distinguished by degree of superior migration from the center of humeral head ro-

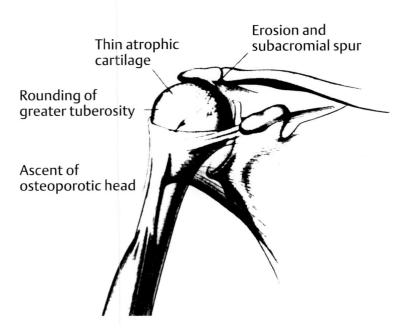

Thin atrophic cartilage

Erosion and subacromial spur

Rounding of greater tuberosity

Ascent of osteoporotic head

Figure 7–1 When pathological changes in cuff tear arthropathy occur, the classic pattern of rotator cuff arthropathy involves the superior migration of an osteoporotic humeral head combined with erosion of the coracoacromial arch. From Neer CS, Craig EV, Fukuda H. Cuff tear arthropathy. J Bone Joint Surg Am 1983; 65: 1236. Adapted by permission.

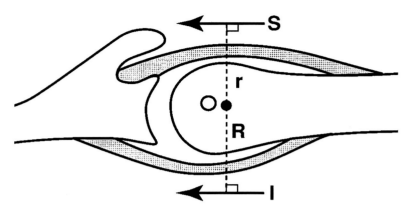

Figure 7–2 The transverse force couple between the subscapularis anteriorly and the external rotators (infraspinatus, teres minor) posteriorly are evident on an axillary view diagram. These two forces balance and centralize (in conjunction with the coronal forces of the deltoid and supraspinatus) the humeral head to produce concavity compression with the glenoid. From Jensen KL, Williams GR, Russell IJ, Rockwood CA Jr. Current concepts review: rotator cuff arthropathy. J Bone Joint Surg Am 1999; 81: 1316. Adapted by permission.

tation and the amount of instability of the center of rotation (see Chapter 6, Fig. 6–3). The proposed benefits of this classification include decision-making for appropriate implant selection, adjustment of reconstruction goals, and assessment of patient functional outcomes.

History and Physical Exam

Patients with RCA are generally in their 7th decade or older and are usually women.[8] In general, a long history of progressive pain, particularly at night is given by the patient. The dominant upper extremity is more commonly involved. Diminished active shoulder motion (abduction, ER) with stiffness during passive range of motion (ROM) exercises is noted. Atrophy of the supraspinatus and infraspinatus muscles with variable degrees of abduction and ER weakness occur. Shoulder swelling may be present secondary to excessive fluid pressure in the subacromial bursa. Aspiration of this fluid may be blood tinged or bloody in appearance. Removal of this fluid combined with steroid and anesthetic injections may provide temporary relief; however, fluid reaccumulation is common.[8-10]

Imaging

True anteroposterior (AP) and axillary lateral views may demonstrate the characteristic radiographic findings of RCA (**Fig. 7–3**),[8-10] Although not necessary, magnetic resonance imaging (MRI) may be helpful in clinical scenarios where physical exam findings are ambiguous or difficult to interpret (i.e., secondary to pain).[8]

Surgical Treatment

Indications

The main impetus for surgical management of RCA is unremitting, progressive pain recalcitrant to nonoperative

measures such as rest, nonsteroidal antiinflammatory medications, corticosteroid injections, ROM exercises, fluid aspiration, and oral analgesics.[8-10]

Contraindications

A denervated or weakened anterior deltoid (less than antigravity strength), incompetent coracoacromial arch, and active or suspected sepsis all preclude implant arthroplasty as a treatment option.[9]

Treatment Options

RCA, as a distinct endpoint along the continuum of glenohumeral degeneration, presents a unique operative challenge to the surgeon. The historical failure of total shoulder arthroplasty with glenoid component loosening, second-

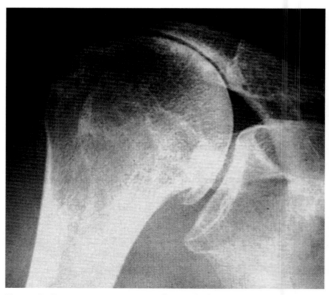

Figure 7–3 An anteroposterior radiograph demonstrates superior humeral head migration with rounding of the greater tuberosity (femoralization) and erosion of the coracoacromial arch (acetabularization).

ary to abnormal shoulder kinematics, precludes its use. Previous alternative attempts at surgical correction for improvements in pain relief, stability, and increased motion with constrained and semiconstrained devices have provided marginal results with unacceptable complication rates.[8–10] Advances in implant design, instrumentation, and surgical technique have propelled further interest in the utilization of these devices, but long-term follow-up is lacking. Short-term results, though promising, still present unacceptable complication rates.[10]

The treatment goals of CTA are similar to those in standard degenerative (osteoarthritis) and inflammatory conditions (rheumatoid arthritis): shoulder arthroplasty should provide pain relief, restore glenohumeral stability, and improve functional motion (i.e., for activities of daily living). Based upon the severity of the arthropathy, the concept of "limited-goals" surgery may be appropriate when evaluating these patients.[11] A current review of the literature indicates that the unconstrained implant (i.e., hemiarthroplasty) design has remained a viable alternative in the treatment of RCA. Utilizing the standard deltopectoral approach, Arntz, Jackins, and Matsen[12] reported their experience with the Neer II prosthesis in the treatment of 19 patients (21 shoulders) over a 9-year period (1978 to 1987). Eighteen shoulders were available for review at a follow-up range of 25 to 122 months. Notably, pain diminished from "marked or disabling" in 14 shoulders to "none or slight" in 10, and "pain with unusual activity" in 4. Active forward elevation improved on average from 66 degrees preoperatively to 109 degrees postoperatively. Hemiarthroplasties were performed only in those patients with a functionally intact coracoacromial arch.[12] Pollock et al[13] in 1992 compared hemiarthroplasty versus total shoulder arthroplasty in 30 shoulders with RC tears. Thirteen shoulders at the time of surgery demonstrated massive irreparable RC tears and were subsequently treated with hemiarthroplasty and cuff débridement. All 12 patients (13 shoulders) reported little or no pain and displayed an average increase of 44 degrees of active forward elevation (average: 64 to 108 degrees) at 41 months postoperatively.

In 1996, Williams and Rockwood[14] reported their results in 20 patients (21 shoulders, average follow-up: 4 years) with irreparable RC tears and glenohumeral arthritis treated with humeral head replacement. Twelve shoulders demonstrated no pain, six were mildly painful, and three were moderately painful. The authors emphasized the need to preserve the coracoacromial ligament if present, and to alter humeral head size to obtain appropriate soft tissue balancing. In the presence of an incompetent coracoacromial arch, some authors have advocated augmentation with iliac crest bone graft or placement of bone from the resected humeral head in the area of the superior glenoid. Such techniques have resulted in noted improvements in pain relief.[8] Recently, Hockman et al[15] underscored the importance of a competent coracoacromial arch with their analysis of anterosuperior restraint in cadaveric specimens with simulated massive RC tears, hu-

meral head replacement, and coracoacromial ligament status. Mean anterosuperior displacement of 3.4 mm occurred in those specimens that underwent coracoacromial ligament release, thus reinforcing its role as a secondary stabilizer to anterosuperior migration in the RC-deficient shoulder. In 1997, Field and colleagues[16] reviewed data on 16 patients who underwent hemiarthroplasty for RCA. Similar to Arntz et al,[12] the surgical technique involved a modular humeral head of appropriate size to allow for articulation with the coracoacromial arch, but to also allow 50% translation on the glenoid surface. The average age of the patient was 74 years and follow-up was at 33 months. With the use of Neer's limited goals criteria, 10 patients were rated as successful and 6 as unsuccessful. Of the six unsuccessful results, 4 patients had previously undergone attempts at RC repair with acromioplasty. Of these 4 patients, 3 demonstrated anterosuperior subluxation after hemiarthroplasty. The authors emphasized the need for good deltoid function, and attributed poor results to prior acromioplasty.[16]

Zuckerman et al[17] performed a retrospective review of 15 shoulders with CTA. With an average patient age of 73 and mean follow-up of 28.2 months, 13 shoulders (13/15, 87%) demonstrated significant improvements in pain relief, with average increases of active forward flexion from 69 to 86 degrees and ER from 15 to 29 degrees. UCLA rating scores improved from 11 to 22 postoperatively.[18] The authors concluded that favorable clinical results may be obtained after hemiarthroplasty.

Sanchez-Sotelo and Cofield presented their review of 33 shoulders (30 patients) managed with hemiarthroplasty in the setting of glenohumeral arthritis with massive, irreparable RC tears.[19] Clinical results were again graded according to the limited-goals criteria of Neer et al.[11] The mean pain scores decreased from 4.2. to 2.2 at most recent follow-up; however, nine shoulders (27%) displayed moderate pain at rest (5 shoulders) or pain with activity (four shoulders). Mean active forward elevation improved from 72 to 91 degrees. Twenty-two shoulders (22/33, 67%) were graded as successful. Of note, anterosuperior instability occurred in seven shoulders associated with a history of subacromial decompression ($p < .04$). The authors concluded that hemiarthroplasty remains a viable and durable option in the treatment of CTA with an intact coracoacromial arch.[19]

Recently, Visotsky et al[6] reported their results utilizing a novel extended humeral head humeral prosthesis (Global Advantage CTA, DePuy Orthopaedics, Inc., Warsaw, IN) for the treatment of CTA.[6] According to the Seebauer classification, nine shoulders were type IA, 28 were type IB, and 23 were type IIA. Average age at the time of surgical intervention was 70.4 years (range: 55 to 89). All patients underwent a deltopectoral approach with preservation of the coracoacromial arch and débridement of residual RC tissue. Average duration of follow-up was 32.4 months (minimum 2 years). At reported follow-up,[20] statistically significant ($p < 0.05$) improvements were observed with Visual Analog

Scale scores (9.3 to 1.9) for pain, average ER (8 to 30 degrees), average forward flexion (56 to 116 degrees), and American Shoulder and Elbow Surgeons (ASES) Scale[22] scores (29 to 79). Despite the promising findings, the authors emphasized that historical results of hemiarthroplasty in CTA were "good but not completely predictable."

Surgical Technique

Here we detail our preferred patient positioning and surgical approach for CTA (DePuy Orthopaedics, Inc., Warsaw, Indiana) hemiarthroplasty in patients with CTA. This extended humeral head prosthesis has a larger area of lateral articulation in abduction and ER when compared with standard humeral heads (**Fig. 7–4**). These steps should be used as guidelines and adjusted to the specific patient. Prior to surgical intervention, regional anesthesia (i.e., interscalene block) may be performed to reduce intraoperative and postoperative pain medication demand. Intravenous antibiotics are administered within 30 minutes of incision. Once general anesthesia has successfully been obtained, the patient is placed in the semi-Fowler position (**Fig. 7–5**) with the head anchored and protected with the McConnell head device (McConnell Orthopedics Inc., Greenville, Texas). Bony landmarks (clavicle, coracoid process, and humerus) are identified. A standard deltopectoral approach is made from the midclavicle medial to the coracoid process to the midhumerus at the deltoid insertion (**Fig. 7–6**). The cephalic vein is identified, protected, and mobilized laterally to maintain continuity with tributaries to the deltoid musculature.

The clavipectoral fascia is incised, and divided from the coracoacromial ligament inferiorly to the upper border of the pectoralis major. A large effusion may be released. If visualization and dislocation maneuvers prove difficult, the upper 1 cm of the pectoralis major tendon may be incised. With sharp and blunt dissection, the subdeltoid and subacromial bursa may be removed. Do not perform an acromioplasty or coracoacromial ligament release because this may compromise postoperative implant stability. The axillary nerve is palpated on the anteroinferior surface of the subscapularis as it traverses posteriorly through the quadrangular space. The biceps tendon may be absent, but if present, is usually attenuated. If intact, we recommend release and tenodesis at the conclusion of the procedure prior to skin closure. The subscapularis is released directly from its humeral insertion and tagged with a 1-mm cottony Dacron suture for later repair through bone tunnels. While protecting the axillary nerve with a Scofield retractor, the anteroinferior capsule is released to approximately the 6 o'clock position. Posteriorly placed Darrach retractors (Specialty Surgical Instrumentation Inc., Huntsville, Alabama) are combined with gentle arm extension to dislocate the humeral head (**Fig. 7–7**). If further difficulty is encountered with exposure, the posterior capsule may be released from its glenoid insertion. RC remnants are excised. Remaining posteroinferior cuff is protected with a modified curved Crego (Wright Medical Inc., Huntsville, Alabama). If the humeral head demonstrates significant collapse, preoperative radiographs of the contralateral shoulder may aid in creating a template of the correct position of the humeral head osteotomy. A special template is utilized to mark the angle

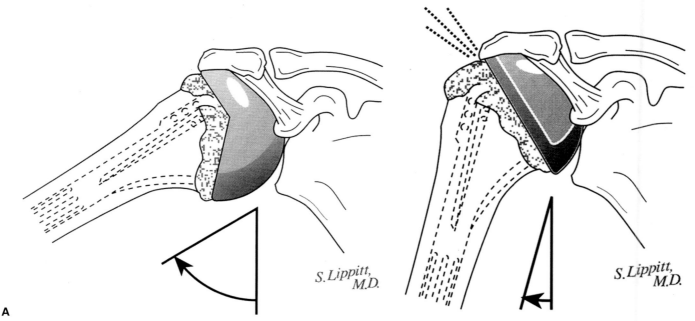

A

B

Figure 7–4 In this Depuy CTA (cuff tear arthropathy; DePuy Orthopaedics, Inc., Warsaw, IN) humeral head implant, greater excursion is noted in **(A)** abduction with an extended lateral humeral head surface when compared with **(B)** a standard humeral head implant. Images appear courtesy of DePuy Orthopaedics, Inc.

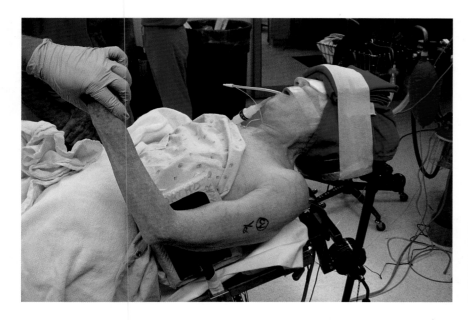

Figure 7–5 This patient is positioned in the semi-Fowler (beach chair) position with the head stabilized with a McConnell head holder (McConnell Orthopedics Inc., Greenville, Texas), thus allowing easy access to the shoulder region and improved ability to dislocate the shoulder.

of head resection. With the humerus parallel to the floor and the arm externally rotated to 30 degrees, the humeral osteotomy is performed with an oscillating saw on power. This single cut removes the head at the appropriate angle and retroversion. The resected head is measured with the available templates and saved for possible bone grafting with final stem implantation.

Axial reamers are introduced into the proximal humerus at the most superolateral aspect of the osteotomy site. Sequential reamers are utilized until cortical contact is obtained. The appropriately sized broach is selected. It

is imperative that the stem not be placed in varus because this will place the humeral head prosthesis in a far medial position, and may result in excessive greater tuberosity resection. Standard trial heads are utilized to assess intraoperative motion and corresponding soft tissue balancing. Peripheral humeral neck osteophytes are removed with an osteotome and rongeur. The humerus is then reduced to assess ROM and stability. With the arm abducted to 90 degrees, internal rotation should be >70 degrees. Posterior translation of the humeral head with the arm in neutral rotation should approach 50% of the glenoid surface.

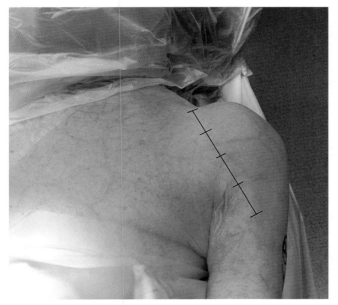

Figure 7–6 Bony landmarks (clavicle, coracoid process, and humerus) are identified, and a standard deltopectoral approach is made from the midclavicle medial to the coracoid process to the midhumerus at the deltoid insertion.

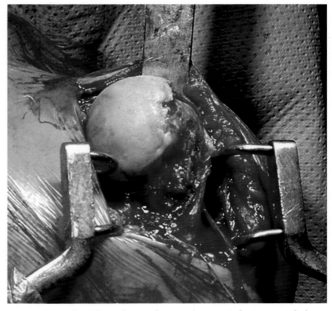

Figure 7–7 After the subscapularis and anteroinferior capsule have been released, the arm is extended to facilitate dislocation of the humeral head. Note the complete absence of the anterosuperior cuff.

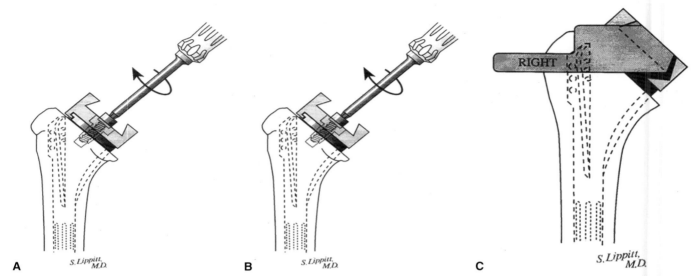

A

B

C

Figure 7–8 (A–C) In a humeral head resection, the side-specific, cuff tear arthropathy cutting guide is applied to the trial broach after soft tissue balancing has been performed with a standard humeral head trial.

If intraoperative motion is suboptimal, the humeral head resection may be lowered in parallel with the original osteotomy with care taken to not violate the posterior cuff. The posterior capsule may be incised to obtain appropriate humeral head excursion. The humeral head is then redislocated, and the trial head is replaced with the CTA head resection guide specific to the left or right humerus (**Fig. 7–8**). An oscillating saw is used to remove bone from the greater tuberosity (**Fig. 7–9**). The jig is removed; the transverse cut is manually completed medially with a rongeur or bur to meet the original oblique neck cut (**Fig. 7–10**). Care must be taken to remove excess bone between the transverse cut and the oblique cut; otherwise, stem orientation and head placement may be affected. An appropriately sized CTA trial head is seated on the trial stem (**Fig. 7–11**). The shoulder is then reduced, and soft tissue balancing is as-

sessed as previously described. The trial head and stem are removed. Drill holes are made in the proximal humerus, approximately one centimeter distal to the osteotomy site. Pass sutures are threaded through these drill holes for later subscapularis repair. If more ER is necessary, 1 cm of medialization of the subscapularis repair will provide ~20 degrees of additional motion. The final implant is assembled on the back table, while autogenous cancellous bone harvested from the resected humeral head is introduced into the proximal metaphyseal region to augment press fit placement of the final implant. The final implant is placed and the shoulder is reduced for subsequent subscapularis repair (**Fig. 7–12**). The wound is thoroughly irrigated with antibiotic solution, and soft tissues are infiltrated with local anesthetic. Two inch drains are placed deep to the deltoid and conjoint tendon. If an interscalene block is not used,

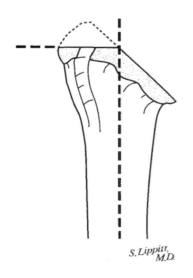

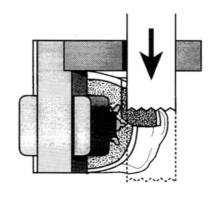

Figure 7–9 In a humeral head resection, an oscillating saw is used to remove bone from the greater tuberosity, taking care not to alter the initial neck osteotomy angle.

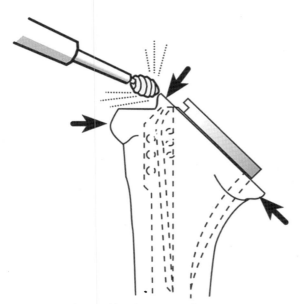

Figure 7–10 In a humeral head resection, the cutting jig is removed, and the transverse cut is completed manually with a rongeur or bur to meet the original oblique neck cut.

we recommend use of a commercially available indwelling pain catheter-pump device placed in similar fashion to the drain. The subcutaneous tissue is closed with 2–0 Vicryl suture (Ethicon, Somerville, New Jersey). The skin is carefully reapproximated with a running subcuticular nylon suture. Sterile dressing is applied; a sling and ice pack are applied for comfort purposes. Prior to patient extubation, intraoperative AP and axillary lateral radiographs are obtained to confirm anatomic reconstruction and to exclude periprosthetic fracture or shoulder dislocation (**Fig. 7–13**).

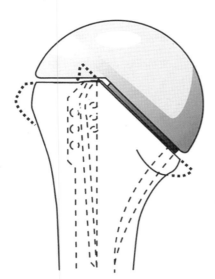

Figure 7–11 In this Depuy CTA (cuff tear arthropathy; DePuy Orthopaedics, Inc., Warsaw, Indiana) trial placement, an appropriately sized CTA trial head is seated on the trial stem with reassessment of intraoperative motion. Image appears courtesy of DePuy Orthopaedics, Inc.

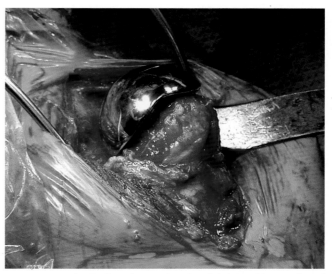

Figure 7–12 The final implant is placed and the shoulder is reduced for subsequent subscapularis repair through bone tunnels.

Postoperative Care and Rehabilitation

On the first postoperative day, instructions to the patient are given regarding passive ROM exercises. Unrestricted passive flexion is obtained with a patient-driven pulley system. Passive ER is performed with a 3-ft stick within limits deemed appropriate by the surgeon and is done in conjunction with pendulum exercises. Patients should perform these exercises 3 to 4 times a day, 7 days a week. The patient is encouraged to use the hand and arm for activities of daily living. Drains and pain pump catheters are generally removed on postoperative day two during the dressing change. Most patients are discharged on the third postoperative day. Sutures are removed at 2 weeks. At 6 weeks, active and active assisted ROM exercises are performed by the patient without restriction. At 3 months, resistance exercises with Therabands (The Hygenic Corp., Akron, Ohio) are used by the patient to strengthen deltoid and RC muscles. Patients should be informed that the rehabilitation process is a lifelong commitment.

Results Analysis

Several of us (JLV, MAW, CAR) conducted a retrospective analysis on 53 (57 shoulders) cases of shoulder hemiarthroplasty with the CTA humeral head prosthesis (DePuy Orthopaedics, Inc., Warsaw, Indiana) performed from 1998 to 2004 for RCA. A standard deltopectoral approach was utilized with appropriate soft tissue balancing as previously described. All patients began passive ROM exercises on postoperative day one. At the time of surgical intervention, all shoulders demonstrated advanced glenohumeral arthritis with complete detachment of the supraspinatus and infraspinatus with variable involvement of the teres minor and subscapularis.

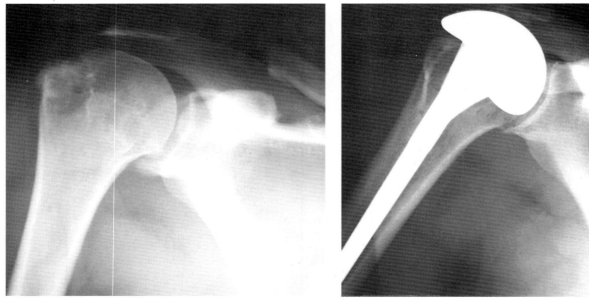

A   B

Figure 7–13 Preoperative films (**A**) confirm cuff tear arthropathy in a patient with progressive shoulder pain refractory to nonoperative measures. Intraoperative x-rays (**B**) document anatomic reconstruction and exclude periprosthetic fracture or shoulder dislocation.

The mean patient age was 69 years (range: 41 to 86), and average follow-up was 25 months (range: 2 to 66). ROM, pain relief (Visual Analog Scale scores), Simple Shoulder Test[21] (SST), and modified American Shoulder and Elbow Surgeons (ASES) scores[22] were assessed preoperatively and postoperatively. On average, active forward elevation increased from 53 to 92 degrees, and active ER increased from 14 to 40 degrees. Visual analog pain scores improved on average from 6.4 to 1.8 (10-point scale). SST and modified ASES scores improved from 2.2 to 6 (out of a possible 12 points), and 29.9 to 63.5 (out of a possible 100), respectively. Salient findings from our study indicate that favorable clinical results may be obtained after hemiarthroplasty for CTA with limited goals criteria.[11]

References

1. Adams R. Illustrations of the Effects of Rheumatic Gout or Chronic Rheumatic Arthritis on All the Articulations. With Descriptive and Explanatory Statements. London: John Churchill and Sons; 1857: 1–31
2. Adams R. A Treatise of Rheumatic Gout of Chronic Rheumatic Arthritis of All the Joints. 2nd ed. London: John Churchill and Sons; 1873:91–175
3. Neer CS II, Craig EV, Fukuda H. Cuff-tear arthropathy. J Bone Joint Surg Am 1983;65:1232–1244
4. Burkhart SS. Fluoroscopic comparison of kinematic patterns in massive rotator cuff tears. A suspension bridge model. Clin Orthop Relat Res 1992;284:144–152
5. Saha AK. Dynamic stability of the glenohumeral joint. Acta Orthop Scand 1971;42:491–505
6. Visotsky JL, Basamania C, Seebauer L, Rockwood CA Jr, Jensen KL. Cuff tear arthropathy: pathogenesis, classification, and algorithm. J Bone Joint Surg Am 2004;86:35–40
7. Seebauer L. Biomechanical classification of cuff tear arthropathy. Abstract presented at: Global Shoulder Society Meeting; July 17–19, 2003; Salt Lake City, UT
8. Zeman CA, Arcand MA, Cantrell JS, Skedros JG, Burkead WZ Jr. The rotator cuff-deficient arthritic shoulder: diagnosis and surgical management. J Am Acad Orthop Surg 1998;6:337–348
9. Collins DN, Harryman DT II. Arthroplasty for arthritis and rotator cuff deficiency. Orthop Clin North Am 1997;28:225–239
10. Bohsali KI, Wirth MA, Rockwood CA Jr. Current concepts review: Complications of total shoulder arthroplasty. J Bone Joint Surg Am 2006;88:2279–2292
11. Neer CS II, Watson KC, Stanton FJ. Recent experience in total shoulder replacement. J Bone Joint Surg Am 1982;64:319–337
12. Arntz CT, Jackins S, Matsen FA III. Prosthetic replacement of the shoulder for the treatment of defects in the rotator cuff and the surface of the glenohumeral joint. J Bone Joint Surg Am 1993;75:485–491
13. Pollock RG, Deliz ED, McIlveen SJ, Flatow EL, Bigliani LU. Prosthetic replacement in rotator cuff-deficient shoulders. J Shoulder Elbow Surg 1992;1:173–186
14. Williams GR Jr, Rockwood CA Jr. Hemiarthroplasty in rotator cuff-deficient shoulders. J Shoulder Elbow Surg 1996;5:362–367
15. Hockman DE, Lucas GL, Roth CA. Role of the coracoacromial ligament as restraint after shoulder hemiarthroplasty. Clin Orthop Relat Res 2004;419:80–82
16. Field LD, Dines DM, Zabinski SJ, Warren RF. Hemiarthroplasty of the shoulder for rotator cuff arthropathy. J Shoulder Elbow Surg 1997;6:18–23
17. Zuckerman JD, Scott AJ, Gallagher MA. Hemiarthroplasty for cuff tear arthropathy. J Shoulder Elbow Surg 2000;9:169–172
18. Ellman H, Hanker G, Bayer M. Repair of the rotator cuff. End result study of factors influencing reconstruction. J Bone Joint Surg Am 1986;6:1136–1144

til it was fully seated against the concave surface. For the Grammont baseplates, the central peg was tapped into the hole until the baseplate was fully seated against the foam block. Both baseplates were further secured with four peripheral screws, including two 3.5-mm diameter by 26-mm long cortical screws and two 4.5-mm diameter by 24-mm long cortical screws. The 3.5-mm screws were inserted at a 90-degree angle and the 4.5-mm diameter screws were inserted at a 60-degree angle relative to the baseplates. Two of the peripheral holes on the Grammont baseplate were threaded to mate with threads on the heads of the 4.5-mm screws. None of the peripheral holes on the RSP baseplate were threaded.

A shear load of 756 N was applied to the rim of each baseplate using a flat plate indenter attached to a servo-hydraulic load apparatus (model 8521, Instron Corp., Canton, MA). This load acted parallel to the baseplate surface with a displacement rate of 150 N/s. Baseplate motion was measured using a digital displacement gauge (model 543–683, Mitutoyo America Corp., Aurora, IL) with a resolution of 10 μm. Baseplate motion was defined as component displacement from 0 N to 756 N loads. Three repetitions were completed for each baseplate.

Results

Baseplate motion was significantly lower for the RSP baseplates at 310 ± 20 μm than the Grammont baseplates at 367 ± 23 μm ($p = 0.016$). Therefore, it was concluded that baseplate motion was significantly lower for reverse shoulder designs using a central cancellous screw and four peripheral cortical screws compared with reverse shoulder designs using a central peg and four peripheral cortical screws.

The attachment of the glenosphere to the baseplate (collectively called the glenoid component) increases the forces at the bone/baseplate junction. The choice of glenosphere also plays a part, as increasing the distance between the glenoid bone and the COR increases the forces seen at the bone/baseplate junction. As mentioned above, initial designs of the RSP were available with two glenosphere choices—the 32-mm neutral glenosphere with a COR (COR) 10-mm outside the glenoid and a 32 - 4 mm glenosphere with a COR 6-mm outside the glenoid. To determine the baseplate micromotion of the entire glenoid component (the glenosphere and the baseplate) with all peripheral screws under physiological loading and the maximum load at failure of fixation, two tests were conducted to determine loads to failure and micromotion during cyclic loading.

First, a servo-hydraulic machine was used to articulate the socket component with the glenosphere. A compressive and shear load was applied while load-displacement output was continuously monitored (**Fig. 8–11**). The tests were continued until a substantial drop in the shear load occurred with increasing displacement. The load to failure for both the RSP and the Grammont design was ~1000 N and not significantly different from each other (**Table 8–3**).

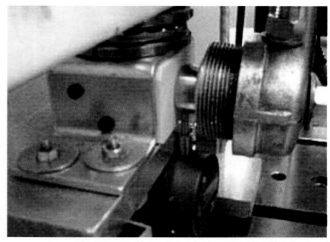

Figure 8–11 A servo-hydraulic machine articulating the socket component with the glenosphere.

Next, a study was conducted to evaluate the initial glenoid component fixation of the three different designs (RSP 32-mm neutral, 32 - 4 mm, and the Grammont 36 mm). Compressive and shear loads were applied to the glenoid components to create eccentric loading conditions similar to the rocking-horse loosening mechanism that has been observed in patients with rotator cuff deficiency treated with a total shoulder prosthesis.[16] This study found that fixation of the two available RSP glenospheres with 3.5-mm screws demonstrated increased baseplate micromotion compared with the Grammont design. However, micromotion for all devices was below 150 μm, which is considered necessary for successful bone ingrowth.[15] The results of this study provided some validation toward the use of RSP glenospheres with more lateral CORs that were fixed with 3.5-mm nonlocking screws.

Based on the above tests, it was apparent that the RSP, despite having a lateral COR, had adequate glenoid fixation. Unfortunately, clinical use of RSP 32-mm neutral and 32 - 4-mm glenospheres with 3.5-mm nonlocking screws resulted in mechanical failure of the baseplate in some of the devices. In total, 267 shoulders were implanted with the RSP between 1998 and 2004 exclusively using the 3.5-mm peripheral screws. Out of these 267 patients, there were 21 baseplate failures (7.8%). Evaluation of two of the initial baseplate failures was performed using scanning electron microscopy.

Scanning Electron Microscopy of Failed Baseplates[17]

Purpose

In an attempt to understand the failure mode of failed glenoid fixation, a retrieval analysis of failed baseplates was conducted.

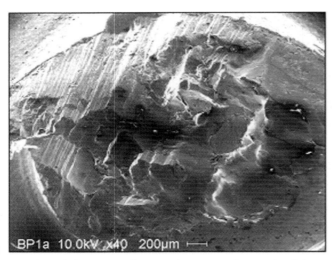

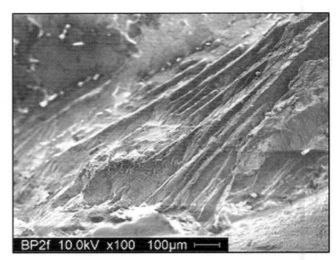

Figure 8–12 (A) Scanning electron microscope micrographs of the center screw, and **(B)** the baseplate undersurface.

Methods

A scanning electron microscope was used to determine if bone ingrowth occurred and to analyze fatigue characteristics at the center screw. Two baseplates were available for analysis.

Results

Minimal bone ingrowth was observed on the porous coating on the undersurface of the baseplate. The striations of the central screw could be accurately characterized as fatigue failure (**Fig. 8–12**).

Conclusion

The findings of these analyses suggest that baseplate failure was a fatigue phenomenon, which resulted in failure of bone ingrowth comparable to fixation failure occurring in nonunions.

Once it was determined that the mode of mechanical failure of the baseplate was fatigue fracture due to lack of bone ingrowth, attempts were made to further improve fixation of the baseplate. The idea of adding peripheral locking screws to provide additional baseplate fixation was conceived and the biomechanical study was repeated using 5-mm locking and nonlocking screws (**Fig. 8–13**).

Screw Fixation of Glenoid Components Using 5.0-mm Screws[18]

Purpose

This study was divided into two experiments. The first experiment measured the baseplate micromotion after varying the screw diameter, screw type, and/or glenosphere

type. The second experiment used an "offset gauge" device to compare baseplate motion within a range of lateral offset magnitudes, using two types of peripheral screws for fixation. Lateral offset was defined as the distance from the glenoid baseplate to the center of articular contact between the glenosphere and the polyethylene cup.

Methods: First Variation

Two variations of the RSP glenosphere (32-mm neutral and 32 - 4 mm) were tested in addition to a 36-mm glenoid component of the Grammont design. These devices had varying lateral offsets, defined as the distance from

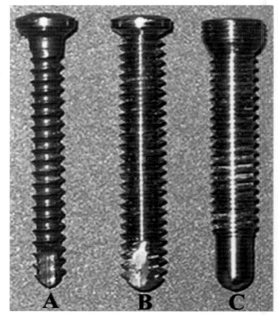

Figure 8–13 (A) 3.5-mm-diameter nonlocking, **(B)** 5.0-mm-diameter nonlocking, or **(C)** 5.0-mm-diameter locking screws.

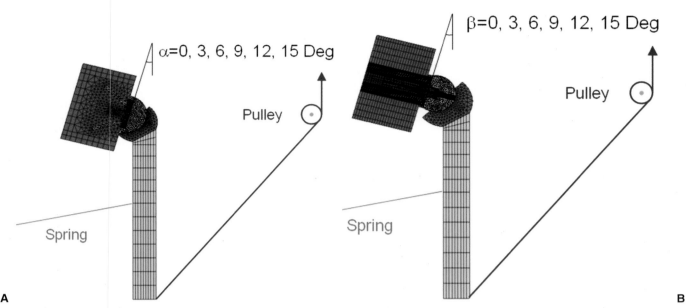

Figure 8–19 Loading system of the three-dimensional finite element model for **(A)** the Grammont design, and **(B)** the Reverse Shoulder Prosthesis.

15 degrees reduces the bone/base-plate relative motions for both the Grammont design and RSP (**Fig. 8–21**).

Radiographic Study of Baseplate and Glenosphere Position[22]

Purpose

The working hypothesis for this study was that patients with mechanical failure of their RSP baseplates were implanted with a more superior tilt than those that did not fail.

Methods

A retrospective review was performed of 203 consecutive patients with a minimum of 2-year follow-up, which were treated with an RSP using the initial baseplate design utilizing 3.5-mm peripheral nonlocking screws. There were 14 patients with mechanical failure of the baseplate (8 men, 6 women) and 189 patients without failure (55 men, 134 women) who were included in the study. To identify the tilt of the baseplate relative to the scapula, the spinospheric angle was established for each patient (**Fig. 8–22**).

Results

The spinospheric angle averaged 72 degrees (Range = 50 to 96 degrees, SD = 8.6 degrees) for the 189 patients without mechanical failure. In the 14 failures, mean spinospheric angle was 80 degrees (Range = 71 to 84 degrees, SD = 5 degrees). A statistically significant difference in spinospheric angle was observed between the failure and nonfailure group ($p = 0.0014$).

The 84-month survival rate for the glenosphere/baseplate construct was 98% in 101 out of 203 patients whose spinospheric angle was 72 degrees or less (Group 1), whereas the survival rate for the other 102 patients whose

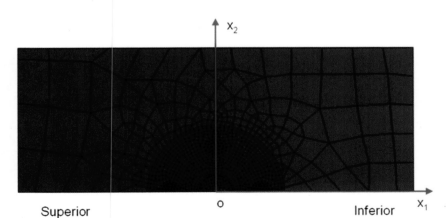

Figure 8–20 Finite Element Analysis coordinate system for recording relative glenosphere motion.

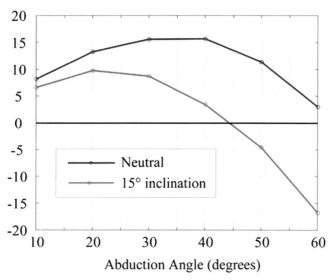

Figure 8–21 Graph demonstrating that inferior tilting of the baseplate with a sufficiently large inclination angle up to 15 degrees reduces the bone/baseplate relative motions for both the Grammont design and the Reverse Shoulder Prosthesis.

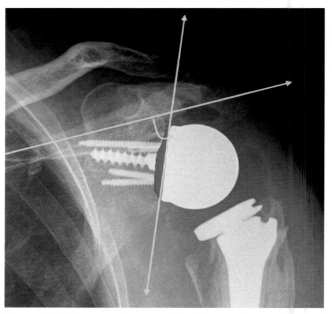

Figure 8–22 The spinospheric angle is defined as the arc subtended by the baseplate and scapular spine in the coronal plane, as seen on the anteroposterior view.

spinospheric angle was greater than 73 degrees (Group 2) was 88% (**Fig. 8–23**).

Conclusion

Superior tilting of the glenosphere/baseplate construct may increase the incidence of mechanical failure and lead to a lower survivability of the implant.

Clearly, implantation of the baseplate in the proper position is essential. Based on the radiographic, biomechanical, and computer modeling studies, the current recommendation is to implant the baseplate with an inferior tilt up to 15 degrees.

The biomechanical modeling and finite element modeling described above were performed utilizing models of good bone, with similar mechanical characteristics to a

normal scapula. However, when similar studies were performed using a poor bone model, neither the Grammont nor RSP design was able to minimize micromotion between the prosthesis and the bone to below 150 μm. Concerns regarding implantation of the RSP design in poor glenoid bone or in situations where the purchase of the center screw was suboptimal resulted in the addition of multiple glenosphere options that could provide a more medial COR. In these scenarios, the improved RSP baseplate fixation could be used in conjunction with a glenosphere with a COR as medial as the glenoid surface. The medial COR would lessen the forces at the bone/baseplate interface, but at the cost of decreased potential ROM. Biomechanical modeling was used to further evaluate these new glenosphere options.

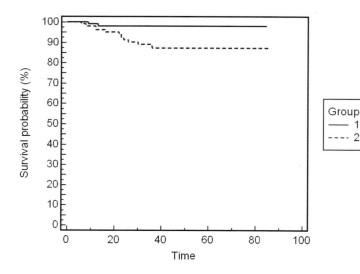

Figure 8–23 Kaplan–Meier survivorship of patients whose spinospheric angle was ≤72 degrees (group 1) and whose spinospheric angle was >73 degrees (group 2).

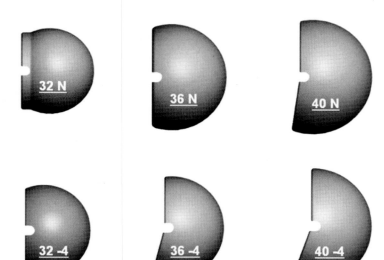

Figure 8–24 Diagram of the different glenospheres available for the Reverse Shoulder Prosthesis. The different glenospheres offer a range of centers of rotation from right at the glenoid (40 mm - 4 mm) to 10 mm lateral to the glenoid (32-mm neutral).

Effect of Changing the Distance Between the Center of Rotation and the Glenoid Surface on Baseplate Fixation[23,24]

Purpose

Due to the increasing options available for RSP glenospheres, a study was developed to quantify the biomechanical differences between them. It was hypothesized that by decreasing the distance from the glenoid surface to the COR, forces at the device–bone interface would decrease.

Methods

The effect of varying the COR on baseplate fixation was evaluated using biomechanical, analytical, and fine element analysis models. Six available RSP glenospheres (**Fig. 8–24**) were used along with the 36-mm Grammont gleno-

sphere. The distance from the glenoid to the COR ranged from 0 mm to 10 mm (**Table 8–5**).

Biomechanical Model

A biomechanical testing apparatus similar to the one discussed above in the study on screw fixation of glenoid components using 5.0-mm screws was used to test each glenosphere implanted in bone models simulating excellent quality glenoid bone. All RSP glenospheres/baseplate combinations were implanted using 5.0-mm locking screws at 90-degree angles relative to the baseplate. The Grammont glenosphere/baseplate combination was implanted with two nonlocking screws placed at 60 degrees relative to the baseplate and two locked screws placed at 90 degrees relative to the baseplate. The micromotion between the baseplate and glenoid bone was measured 3-mm away from the bone/baseplate interface after an application of 1000 cycles of shear loading at 756 N or one times body weight.

Table 8–5   Differences in Dimensions for the Various Reverse Glenospheres Used in This Study

Glenosphere	R (mm)	h_1 (mm)	h_2 (mm)	h_3 (mm)	h_0 (mm)
RSP (40 mm - 4 mm)	20	−3	3	0	20
Grammont (36 mm)	18	−2	3	1	19
RSP (36 mm - 4 mm)	18	−1	3	2	20
RSP (40-mm neutral)	20	1	3	4	24
RSP (36-mm neutral	18	3	3	6	24
RSP (32 mm - 4 mm)	16	3	3	6	22
RSP (32-mm neutral)	16	7	3	10	26

Abbreviations: R, glenosphere radius; h_0, distance between the glenoid and the tip of the glenosphere; h_1, distance between the top of the baseplate and the center of rotation; h_2, height of the baseplate; h_3, distance between the glenoid and the center of rotation; RSP, Reverse Shoulder Prosthesis.

Finite Element Analysis

A 3-D axi-symmetric finite element model was created to simulate the mechanical testing described above (**Fig. 8–25**). The finite element setup was modified to change the coefficient of friction between the glenosphere and the socket and to simulate the effect of misalignment between the bone and baseplate.

Analytical Model

A mathematical equation was derived to help predict the effect of changing the coefficient of friction and the distance between the glenoid and the COR on the reaction moment at the bone/baseplate interface at various abduction angles.

Results

The analytical, biomechanical and finite model had close agreement (**Table 8–6**). In vitro mechanical testing indicated that the average baseplate motion during 1000 load cycles ranged from 90 μm to 120 μm for the seven different glenosphere types (**Table 8–7**). Although there was a general trend toward increased baseplate motion with increasing distance from the glenoid to the COR, no significant difference was observed. Static equilibrium analysis found that the reaction moment at the bottom of the baseplate rises monotonically as the coefficient of friction of the articulating surfaces increases and as the distance from the glenoid to the COR increases. Results from the finite element analysis were strongly correlated (Spearman's rank order correlation $\rho_s = 0.829$ and $p = 0.0423$) with the in vitro mechanical testing[25] and confirmed that baseplate motion varied 30 μm or less over the range of glenosphere component sizes tested (**Table 8–7**). Additionally, the finite element analysis found

that a misalignment of 1 degree between the baseplate and the bone axis can lead to micromotion as large as 310 μm and that there is more baseplate motion with a frictional articulating interface than with a smooth contact between the glenosphere and the socket.

Conclusion

Evaluation of data from the mechanical analysis found that despite large differences in distance between the glenoid and the centers of rotation for various glenospheres (0 to 10 mm), the differences in baseplate micromotion from physiological loads in healthy bone is insignificant provided that adequate initial fixation is achieved. The presence of increasing frictional torque increases baseplate micromotion. Additionally, excessive baseplate motion occurs if there is a mismatch between the glenoid and baseplate. It must be noted that smaller reaction moments were seen in the analytical model with centers of rotation closer to the glenoid surface. Therefore, a medial COR may provide the best scenario when confronted with bone deficiency of the glenoid so that forces at the bone/baseplate junction can be minimized.

The addition of locking screws combined with a selection of glenospheres with varying distances from the COR to the glenoid surface (0, 2, 4, 6, and 10 mm) have been used by my practice since January 2004. Additional features of the RSP baseplate aid in achieving stable fixation and promoting bone ingrowth such as the concave baseplate and hydroxyapatite coating on the undersurface. After these changes and up until the time this chapter was being finalized in late 2007, there had been no glenoid-sided mechanical failures.

In the setting of deficient glenoid bone, the current recommendation for establishing stable baseplate fixa-

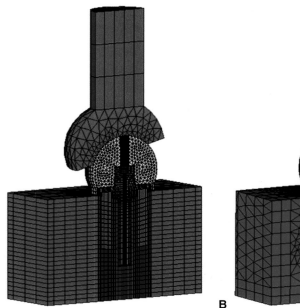
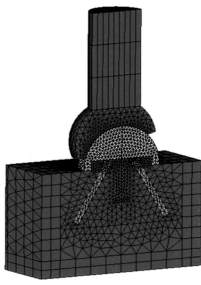

A   B

Figure 8–25 Finite element models for **(A)** the Reverse Shoulder Prosthesis 32-mm neutral, and **(B)** the Grammont 36 mm.

Table 8–6   Comparison of Three Different Modes of Analysis Used in This Study

	Lowest to Highest Baseplate Motion From Mechanical Testing After 1000 cycles of loading	Lowest to Highest Baseplate Motion From Finite Element Analysis at either of the 2 tested coefficients of friction, regardless of where the measurement was taken or the coverage area stimulated	Lowest to Highest Reaction Moment From Static Equilibrium Analysis at $\mu > 0$ and any abduction angle above 0 degrees	
↑ Increasing baseplate micromotion or reaction moment ↓	Grammont (1)	Grammont (1)	RSP 40 minus 4 (0)	↑ Decreasing baseplate micromotion or reaction moment
	RSP 40 neutral (4)	RSP 40 minus 4 (0)	Grammont (1)	
	RSP 40 minus 4 (0)	RSP 36 minus 4 (2)	RSP 36 minus 4 (3)	
	RSP 36 minus 4 (2)	RSP 40 neutral (4)	RSP 40 neutral (4)	
	RSP 32 minus 4 (6)	RSP 32 minus 4 (6)	RSP 32 minus 4 (6)	
	and RSP 32 neutral (10)	RSP 36 neutral (6)	RSP 36 neutral (6)	
	RSP 36 neutral (6)	RSP 32 neutral (10)	RSP 32 neutral (10)	

$\rho_2 = 0.829$
$p = 0.0423$

$\rho_2 = 0.964$
$p = 0.0182$

$\rho_2 = 0.757$
$p = 0.0638$

*Distances between the simulated bone and the centers of rotation of the glenospheres in mm are given in parentheses. The Spearman rank-order correlation coefficient (ρ_s), indicative of the strength of the correlation between the rankings, is given comparing the three analyses. Also, *p*-values give the probability of the derived ρ_s values occurring by chance.
Abbreviation: RSP, Reverse Shoulder Prosthesis.

Table 8–7   Comparison of Baseplate Micromotion between the Finite Element (FE) Analysis and In-Vitro Mechanical Testing

	Distance between simulated glenoid and center of rotation (mm)	Baseplate micromotion measured 3 mm away from the simulated bone/baseplate interface at $\mu = 0$ from FE analysis (μm)	Baseplate micromotion measured 3 mm away from the simulated bone/baseplate interface at $\mu = 0.22$ from FE analysis (μm)	Baseplate micromotion from mechanical testing— 1000 cycles of repetitive shear load (μm)	Difference between FE analysis at $\mu = 0.22$ and mechanical testing
RSP (40 mm - 4 mm)	0	59	74	100 ± 10	26%
Delta-III	1	57	69	90 ± 24	23%
RSP (36 mm - 4 mm)	2	64	77	107 ± 15	28%
RSP (40 mm neutral)	4	69	84	97 ± 12	13%
RSP 36- mm neutral)	6	74	87	120 ± 10	28%
RSP (32 mm - 4 mm)	6	74	86	113 ± 12	24%
RSP (32- mm neutral)	10	84	96	113 ± 6	15%

Abbreviation: RSP, Reverse Shoulder Prosthesis.

tion was developed from a clinical review of RSPs placed in deficient glenoid bone stock. The placement of the central screw in the bone at the junction of the spine of the scapula and the body resulted in consistently strong screw purchase. The bone at the base of the scapula spine was robust, even in the most clinically dire circumstance. We currently recommend placement of the baseplate into this particular location, using 5.0-mm peripheral locking screws, and a glenosphere with a more medial COR.

Humeral-Sided Complications

Initial concerns using the RSP centered on glenoid-sided complications. Clinical experience coupled with basic science research increased the understanding of how to avoid these problems, and has helped to limit their incidence. We now turn our attention to the humeral-sided complications.

The increased constraint of the reverse design places greater force on the humeral side than is typically seen in a conventional total shoulder arthroplasty. In a multicenter study using the Grammont design, a 20% incidence of humeral-sided complications was noted.[26] Humeral complications included in this review were humeral fractures, prosthetic dissociation, prosthetic subsidence, loosening, and radiolucent lines.

The early experience using the RSP noted humeral complications, which were identified during the early clinical trials. Biomechanical models were thus created to gain further understanding as to why these complications occurred and develop solutions to limit these problems in the future.

Polyethylene Disassociation

The initial humeral design used an all polyethylene socket, which was attached to a small metal button (similar to a patellar metal insert in a total knee). The metal button provided a Morse taper attachment to the humeral stem, which could then be cemented. Using this design, there were four cases of polyethylene failure related to disassociation. All of these failures occurred in the revision setting where proximal humeral bone support was deficient, allowing the polyethylene to remain unsupported. The incidence of polyethylene disassociation in the revision setting was thus 3.5% (4/115 revisions). This led to several experiments to test the failure strength of this attachment site.

Mechanical Testing of Proximal Polyethylene Inserts in the Encore Reverse Shoulder Prosthesis

To determine the optimal configuration of the polyethylene component for the RSP, testing was done to determine

the load required to dissociate the polyethylene socket from its metal underside when subjected to a cantilever load. Nine different configurations of polyethylene/metal underside combinations were tested (**Fig. 8–26**), two of which had a screw that improved the fixation between the metal underside and the polyethylene. In all cases, the stem was assembled in a vise fixture. The poly socket and metal backing were connected to the stem and the stem was positioned and clamped into place. A load cell was used to measure the force applied to the poly socket and this load was applied to the polyethylene socket until the polyethylene disassociated from the metal underside. This test helped us determine that the best polyethylene/metal backing combination to use in designs of the RSP should include a screw to better secure the metal backing to the polyethylene component.

Another test was done with the same nine configurations of the socket to determine the number of cycles it would take to cause failure. One humeral stem and one glenoid head were used for all testing. Only the humeral sockets were changed between tests because they were

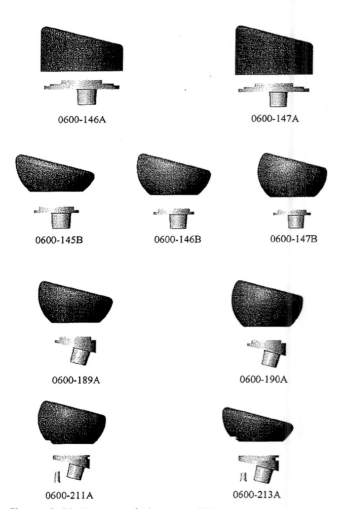

Figure 8–26 Diagram of the nine different configurations of polyethylene/metal backing combinations that were tested.

the only components that were damaged from the fatigue cycling. The fatigue load was applied to the center of the glenoid head, and parallel to the humeral stem. A universal joint was at the bottom so that the humeral stem and socket may deflect in any direction. Testing was continued to failure or 5 million cycles, and then testing was stopped. The failure mode of the humeral sockets was similar to failure experienced when the ultrahigh molecular weight polyethylene socket pulled away from the metal underside at the back of the "U" channel.

After the above testing sequence, the most stable polyethylene insert was selected and was used clinically from 2000 to 2004. Unfortunately, disassociation with the above design still occurred, particularly when there was proximal humeral bone loss. Thus a metal shell encasing the polyethylene socket was added to the design. The purpose of the metal shell was to provide a more secure attachment of the polyethylene socket to the humeral stem and to allow an easy interchange between various sized modular inserts. With this new design, there was a possibility of the polyethylene liner disassociating from the metal shell. Three mechanical tests were performed to evaluate the likelihood of component dissociation. They included (1) the push-out strength of the polyethylene liner relative to the metal shell. This test determined the push-out load required to cause movement between the poly liner and metal shell of the RSP. (2) The torsional load required to cause movement between the poly liner and metal shell. This test was used to determine the force needed to cause the antirotation tabs to shear. (3) The lever-out load required to cause movement between the poly liner and metal shell. This test was used to determine the force needed to cause the poly insert to rock out of the shell.

Currently, the RSP is only available with the polyethylene humeral socket with the metal shell. The metal shell is especially useful in cases with proximal humeral bone loss. Additional investigation of how to provide the best solution to restore proximal humeral bone loss is ongoing. Clinical research suggests that restoration of this bone with an allograft may provide fewer complications such as dislocation and humeral loosening. Currently, biomechanical work is being performed to design an adaptable prosthetic solution for proximal humeral bone loss, which may be less technically challenging and more cost effective than using a bone allograft.

Instability

Cases of dislocation have been reported using the reverse designs, and is often considered the most frequent complication.[27] Reports of the Grammont design note dislocation rates of up to 30%.[28] To further understand potential causes of instability, a multidisciplinary team of scientists developed biomechanical models that could provide further insight into instability of the reverse designs.

Design factors inherent to each of the prostheses directly influence the stability of the implant. These factors play an important role in proper implant selection in cases where stability is a concern. These factors also influence the degree of soft tissue tensioning necessary to keep the device stable. Previous studies on the stability of cadaveric shoulders and total shoulder arthroplasty noted that stability is related to the angle between the radius of curvature of the humeral head and the radius of curvature of the glenoid cavity. As the glenoid cavity becomes deeper and more constrained, the force necessary to dislocate the humeral head increases.[29-41]

Based on this concept, glenospheres with different diameters and sockets depths were developed. To discover how much implant stability can be improved by these geometric changes in prosthetic design, several biomechanical experiments were performed.

Stability

Purpose

The purpose of this study[62] was to quantify the stability of six configurations of the RSP and the Grammont design using experimental and analytical methods.

Methods

Each device was placed into a custom load fixture (**Fig. 8–27**). Two levels of normal force were applied to the humeral component. The peak translational force required to dislocate the glenosphere from the polyethylene socket was measured. Analytical calculations were made to verify the data generated in the experimental part of the experiment.

Results

Forces required for dislocation of the joint were higher for devices with deeper sockets and larger diameter glenospheres. The Grammont design, which has a shallower (8.24 mm) socket, required 172 (±3.19) and 343 (±4.10) N under 111 and 222 N of compressive force, respectively. Under the same compressive forces, dislocation for the 40-mm semiconstrained, the deepest RSP (12.51 mm), required 344 (±10.9) and 532 (±9.25) N. Analytical data correlated well with experimental data, with errors ranging from 2.2 to 25.9% for the 111 N compressive force and from 0.5 to 7.9% for the 222 N compressive force.

Conclusions

Based on the results of this study, an implant with a deeper socket and a larger glenosphere diameter can provide improved stability.

In cases of dislocation, it has been helpful to increase the size of the glenosphere or to use a deeper, semicon-

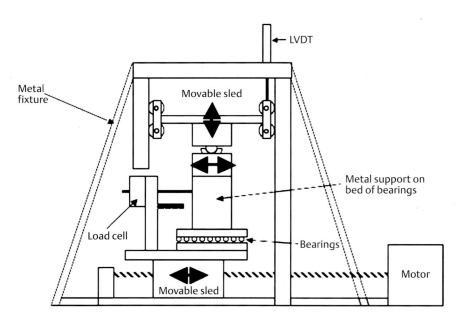

Figure 8–27 Custom apparatus used to measure the force of dislocation of the various glenosphere and socket combinations.

strained socket. The information from the above study has since been used clinically to treat the 7 patients that developed instability after RSP. All 7 patients were revised to a reverse prosthesis with a larger diameter glenosphere and deeper socket. Six of the 7 patients have remained stable after this revision, with one patient developing recurrent instability even after reconstruction. Loss of motion was felt to be related to earlier impingement that occurred with larger glenospheres and deeper sockets. This balance of stability versus mobility was the impetus for additional biomechanical studies to determine the potential variation in glenohumeral motion that occurs with design variations between components.

Range of Motion

Currently, several different prosthetic designs of the reverse shoulder arthroplasties are available in a variety of geometries. Differences in ROM, stability, security of fixation, and motor function may vary among the different implant geometries, so selection of the appropriate shoulder prosthesis requires a priori understanding of the implant geometry.

Few clinical or biomechanical studies have characterized glenohumeral motion associated with reverse shoulder prostheses. Utilizing dynamic radiographs, Seebauer and associates studied isolated glenohumeral elevation following Delta III reverse shoulder implant surgery, and in a cohort of 35 primary and 22 revision patients found active glenohumeral elevation was a maximum of 53 degrees.[5,30] Utilizing a cadaver model, Nyffeler and associates reported that significant improvements in glenohumeral elevation (abduction ROM) could be obtained by altering the position of the Delta III glenosphere more distally on the glenoid.[31] From a clinical standpoint, maximizing the

potential ROM is a key element for functional gains that may be achieved with reverse shoulder prosthetic designs. To further characterize the amount of glenohumeral motion that could be achieved with each design, a Sawbones (Pacific Research Laboratories, Vashon, WA) shoulder model was developed to test motion achieved after implantation of each design.

Range of Motion of the Reverse Shoulder Prosthesis

Purpose

The purpose of this study[61] was to determine differences in abduction ROM (ROM) of six configurations of the RSP. The hypothesis is that the glenohumeral ROM (abduction) is dependent on the COR offset of the glenosphere relative to the glenoid.

Methods

An apparatus was developed to simulate abduction of the humerus in the scapular plane. (**Fig. 8–28**) An orthopedic surgeon implanted six configurations of the RSP into a large left Sawbones scapula and humerus, and ROM data was gathered.

Results

Results showed a positive linear correlation between abduction ROM and COR offset relative to the glenoid. As the COR is moved more lateral from the glenoid, abduction ROM increases. The greatest total abduction ROM was 97 degrees (SD = 0.9) with an RSP glenosphere that has a COR

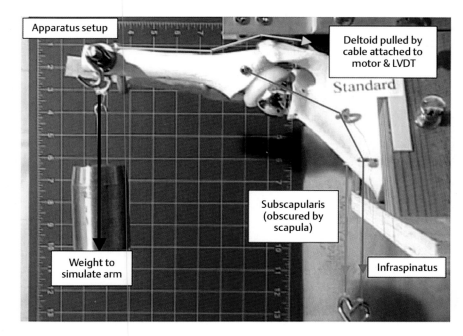

Figure 8–28 Apparatus used to simulate abduction of the humerus in the scapular plane. LVDT, linear variable displacement transducer.

offset of 10 (SD = 0.4) mm from the glenoid and the smallest abduction ROM was 67 degrees (SD = 1.8) with an RSP glenosphere that has a COR offset of 0.5 (SD = 0.1) mm from the glenoid surface.

Conclusions

Improvements in ROM were found to correlate statistically with increased distance from the glenoid to the COR of the glenosphere. CORs that are farther away from the scapula allow the proximal humerus and humeral socket more clearance before impinging on the acromion or superior glenoid, thus maximizing glenohumeral abduction (**Fig. 8–29**). In adduction, a more lateral COR ensures that the medial neck of the prosthesis does not impinge on the inferior aspect of the scapula. This decreases the risk of inferior scapular erosion, and improves overall abduction ROM. Because altered glenohumeral geometry has been shown to affect shoulder muscle forces during abduction,[32] additional work is needed to determine how changes in the COR offset relative to the glenoid may influence shoulder muscle function.

Muscle Function

To understand how muscular function is affected by prosthetic geometric differences, several different biomechanical studies were performed. As mentioned in Chapter 1, the mechanical efficiency of the muscle in generating torque around the joint is determined by the moment arm. Using the direct method, moment arms may be calculated for each joint position by measuring the shortest distance from the action of the muscles to the COR of the joint. The greater the moment arm for each muscle, the greater the

force generated. This approach was undertaken with the various glenospheres described in the above studies, each with a different COR and different radius of curvature. Moment arms were calculated for the deltoid, subscapularis, and infraspinatus, to determine if certain prosthetic geometries are more effective in restoring different types of motion (i.e., greater improvement in rotation than abduction in the scapular plane).

Deltoid Force Comparison Between Glenospheres with Lateralized and Medialized Center of Rotation– Direct Method

Purpose

The purpose of this study was to determine the differences in moment arms of the infraspinatus, subscapularis, and deltoid muscles when different reverse shoulder implants are used.

Methods

Six different configurations of the RSP and the 36-mm Grammont were compared with a hemiarthroplasty. This investigation employed two different procedures: (1) moment arms measured directly from digital video taken of each of the specified muscles while undergoing 90 degrees of scapular abduction, and (2) using a mathematical model to predict deltoid force necessary to abduct the arm through 90 degrees of scapular plane abduction. This was based on a free body diagram generated by biomechanical video analysis.

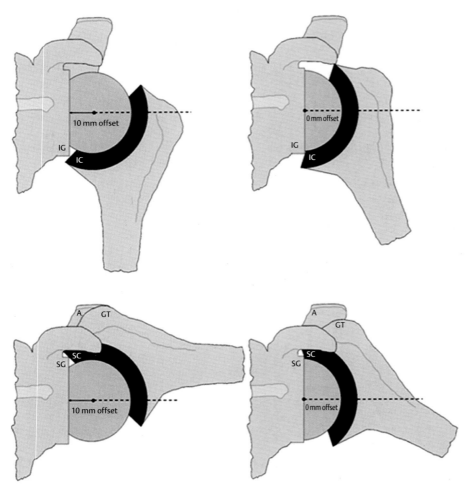

Figure 8–29 Schematic illustration showing the concept of limitations to isolated glenohumeral motion as a consequence of impingement for adduction range of motion (ROM; A1 and B1) and abduction ROM (A2 and B2). Same size glenosphere diameter (32 mm) and different glenosphere COR offset – 10 mm offset (A1 and A2) and 0 mm offset (B1 and B2) – are compared by ROM and prosthetic impingement points. A, Acromion; GT, greater tuberosity; SG, superior glenoid; IG, inferior glenoid; SC, superior cup; IC, inferior cup. ROM shown in illustration does not include scapular motion. Note, for abduction, impingement may occur on superior glenoid (shown) or acromion. (Illustration does not represent experimental data).

An apparatus was developed to simulate abduction of the humerus through 90 degrees (**Fig. 8–30**). A movable sled with a 500-pound load cell (Model LCH-500, OMEGA Engineering Inc., Stamford, CT) was connected via a cable to the attachment site of the deltoid on a simulated humerus. The angle of abduction (± 0.01 degrees) was measured via an electronic goniometer (Greenleaf Medical, Palo Alto, CA) attached via a ring that moves with the humerus. Weights were used to apply a constant force of 60 N to the subscapularis, infraspinatus and, where applicable, the supraspinatus. A weight of 12 N was attached off the end of the humerus to simulate the weight of the arm. Silicone spray was used in the joint to simulate synovial fluid.

Seven different reverse shoulder glenospheres (32-mm neutral, 32 – 4-mm), 36-mm neutral, 36 – 4-mm, 40-mm neutral, and 40 – 4-mm and the 36-mm Grammont design glenosphere were attached to a left Sawbones shoulder model. A hemiarthroplasty was also used to simulate the normal anatomic condition. All configurations were implanted by an orthopedic surgeon using appropriate surgical techniques. Three different Sawbones models were used for each different baseplate configuration and three runs were performed per configuration. Data was collected using a custom-made LABview (National Instruments, Austin, TX) graphical interface, and gathered information on the angle of humeral abduction and force at the origin of the cable. Statistical analysis was performed using a one-way ANOVA and a Student's t test.

Results

Results showed an antagonistic behavior (adductors) of the infraspinatus and the subscapularis in the first 60 degrees of abduction (maximum adductor moment arms of 23.27 mm and 25.21 mm, respectively), then becoming agonist (abductors) to the deltoid the remaining 30 degrees (maximum abductor moment arms of 4.64 mm and 5.87 mm, respectively). This is illustrated by decreasing moment arms to 60 degrees as the line of action of the muscle crosses the COR of the devices and then increasing again as they pass the COR toward the end of 90 degrees of abduction (**Table 8–8**). The trends in the mathematical model correlated well with the biomechanical data and may prove clinically useful for predicting optimal configurations of offset and head size based on bone quality and rotator cuff status.

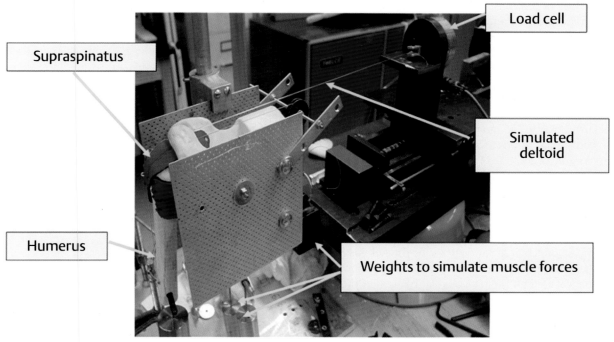

Figure 8–30 Apparatus used to simulate abduction of the humerus through 90 degrees.

Conclusion

Deltoid moment arms are increased in glenospheres with a lateralized COR. Results indicate a possible benefit in using a reduced lateral offset head RSP when deltoid function is compromised.

Additionally, an indirect method of determining the instantaneous moment arm for a given muscle or mechanical advantage with a given glenosphere can be related to the tendon excursion and the joint rotation.

Table 8–8 Moment Arms Calculated In Abduction Using the Origin-Insertion Method (Direct)

	Maximum moment arm origin/insertion method		
	Infraspinatus	Deltoid	Subscapularis
32 Neutral	19.61	47.91	18.98
32 mm - 4 mm	17.93	47.45	20.77
36-mm neutral	23.27	48.99	24.17
36 mm - 4 mm	21.11	46.41	23.57
40-mm Neutral normal	19.48	43.03	22.91
40 mm - 4 mm Normal	20.56	47.34	23.31
40 mm Neutral reduced	20.12	47.36	21.18
40 mm - 4 mm Reduced	21.17	47.19	23.27
Grammont	18.08	41.84	17.65

Indirect Measure of Determining the Instantaneous Moment Arm

Purpose

This study was undertaken to determine differences in shoulder muscle function in reverse implants of various designs when compared with the previously mentioned direct method.

Methods

Measurements were made using six different designs of the RSP, a 36-mm Grammont design and a hemiarthroplasty when implanted into a left Sawbones humerus. The excursion length of the infraspinatus, subscapularis, and middle deltoid were measured while the humerus was rotated through internal and external rotation, as well as elevated through abduction in the scapular plane. Videos were taken of each muscle, and moment arms were measured from the videos using an image processing and analysis program (ImageJ, National Institutes of Health, Bethesda, Maryland).

Results

Deltoid moment arms increased throughout the range of abduction to a maximum of 49.7 ± 1.07 mm for the RSPs, 41.8 ± 0.40 mm for the Grammont design and 26.7 ± 1.61 mm for the hemiarthroplasty. When looking at muscle function during abduction in the subscapularis and infraspinatus, their function changed from adductors to abductors when they crossed the COR of the construct. The moment arms for the subscapularis went from a maximum of 25.2 ± 0.42 mm in adduction at 0 degrees to a maximum of 5.87 ± 1.01 mm in abduction at 90 degrees for the RSPs, a maximum of 17.65 ± 1.35 mm in adduction at 0 degrees to a maximum of 3.2 ± 1.64 mm in abduction at 90 degrees for the Grammont design and a maximum of 5 ± 0.35 mm in adduction at 40 degrees to a maximum of 1.07 ± 0.62 mm in abduction at 90 degrees for the hemiarthroplasty. The moment arms for the infraspinatus followed similar trends as the subscapularis: They went from a maximum of 23.3 ± 0.33 mm in adduction at 0 degrees to a maximum of 4.64 ± 0.34 mm in abduction at 90 degrees for the RSPs, a maximum of 18.1 ± 0.26 mm in adduction at 0 degrees to a maximum of 1.65 ± 0.47 mm in abduction at 90 degrees for the Grammont design and a maximum of 5.53 ± 0.98 mm in adduction at 0 degrees to a maximum of 3.2 ± 0.72 mm in abduction at 90 degrees for the hemiarthroplasty. When looking at internal–external rotation, moment arms were measured for the total angular rotation of the infraspinatus and subscapularis. The maximum moment arms were 36.1 ± 1.27 mm and 31.9 ± 0.43 mm, respectively, for the RSPs, 24.3 ± 0.91 mm and 28.6 ± 1.81 mm, respectively, for the Grammont design, and 23.5 ± 1.30 mm and 26.7 ± 1.38 mm, respectively, for the hemiarthroplasty.

Conclusion

All reverse designs showed similar linear increases in moment arms throughout the range of abduction. This contrasted with the trends in the hemiarthroplasty. The moment of the subscapularis and infraspinatus changes from abduction to adduction as the arm elevates above the prosthetic COR. The greater moment arms of the RSP in internal and external rotation demonstrate a mechanical advantage in having the COR lateral to the glenoid.

To validate these biomechanical studies, a clinical study was established to characterize the functional improvements seen after treatment with the reverse design. A Biodex System 2 dynometer (Biodex Medical Systems, Shirley, NY) study was undertaken to determine the range-specific strength for a group of patients who received an RSP.

Range-Specific Strength after Reverse Shoulder Prosthesis[33]

Purpose

Our goal in this study was to develop a standardized method of measuring shoulder strength during various shoulder motions before and after implantation of the RSP.

Methods

Beginning March 2004, a prospective analysis of shoulder strength was performed in patients who underwent a RSP.

We studied 28 patients who were available for a minimum of 6-month Biodex follow-up. The average age of this study group was 71 years (56 to 86) and included 6 men and 22 women. In terms of pathology, 21 out of 28 had a RSP for primary cuff tear arthropathy and seven out of 28 had RSP to replace a failed hemiarthroplasty done for fracture. Preoperative strength measurements were made using a Biodex dynamometer (Biodex Medical Systems, Shirley, NY) in the sitting position. Postoperative comparisons were made using data at a minimum of 6-month follow-up. Maximum isometric shoulder flexion strength was assessed at four angles of humeral forward elevation: 0, 30, 60, and 90 degrees. Maximum external and internal rotation strengths were also assessed at 0 degrees of abduction and forward elevation.

Results

At 0 degrees of humeral elevation, maximal shoulder flexion strength significantly improved from 7.9 J to 15.0 J ($p = 0.0006$). At 30 degrees of humeral elevation, maximal shoulder flexion strength significantly improved from 3.5 J to 7.7 J ($p = 0.042$). At 60 degrees of humeral elevation, maximal shoulder flexion strength improved from 3.2 J to 4.9 J, and at 90 degrees, maximal shoulder flexion strength improved from 2.8 J to 4.4 J. Neither the improvements at 60 degrees or at 90 degrees were significant ($p = 0.52$ and $p = 0.57$, respectively). Internal rotation strength significantly improved from 10.5 J preoperatively to 14.9 J postoperatively and external rotation strength significantly improved from 7.4 preoperatively to 10.8 postoperatively ($p = 0.031$ and $p = 0.007$, respectively).

Conclusion

The RSP may significantly improve isometric forward flexion strength at 0 and 30 degrees of humeral elevation. Additionally, significant improvements of internal and external rotation strength were seen. Further research is necessary to understand the impact of prosthetic design on muscle strength and function following reverse arthroplasty.

Conclusion

The RSP provides a viable option to restore motion and relieve pain in patients with CTA who have few other options. The design of the RSP was inspired by Grammont's design, but with the advantage of keeping the COR lateral to the glenoid, as it is in the normal shoulder. The RSP design provides the option of a lateral COR which can increase potential ROM at the shoulder joint, improve rotational strength, avoid scapula notching, and maintain deltoid contour. The forces at the bone-baseplate junction may increase; however, with adequate fixation, bone ingrowth can be achieved. In cases of glenoid bone deficiency or suboptimal center screw purchase, a glenosphere with a medial COR can be selected.

Complications on both the humeral and glenoid side have occurred, many of which have been related to design features and technical errors in placement of the prosthesis. Further biomechanical studies are needed to better understand the effect of soft tissue tension and other factors, which may affect the final outcome in patients who are treated with the Reverse Shoulder Prosthesis. The reverse shoulder design will continue to evolve as our understanding of the mechanics of the prosthesis improves.

References

1. Bayley JIL, Kessel L. The Kessel total shoulder replacement. In: Bayley I, Kessel L, eds. Shoulder Surgery. New York: Springer-Verlag; 1982:160–164
2. Boileau P, Watkinson DJ, Hatzidakis AM, Balg F. Grammont reverse prosthesis: design, rationale, and biomechanics. J Shoulder Elbow Surg 2005; 14(1, Suppl S)147S–161S
3. Delloye C, Joris D, Colette A, Eudier A, Dubuc JE. Mechanical complications of total shoulder inverted prosthesis. Rev Chir Orthop Reparatrice Appar Mot 2002;88(4):410–414
4. Werner CM, Steinmann PA, Gilbart M, Gerber C. Treatment of painful pseudoparesis due to irreparable rotator cuff dysfunction with the Delta III reverse-ball-and-socket total shoulder prosthesis. J Bone Joint Surg Am 2005;87(7):1476–1486
5. Seebauer L. Reverse prosthesis through a superior approach for cuff tear arthropathy. Tech Shoulder Elbow Surg 2006;7(1):13–26
6. Sirveaux F, Favard L, Oudet D, Huquet D, Walch G, Mole D. Grammont inverted total shoulder arthroplasty in the treatment of glenohumeral osteoarthritis with massive rupture of the cuff. Results of a multicentre study of 80 shoulders. J Bone Joint Surg Br 2004;86(3):388–395
7. Nyffeler RW, Werner CM, Simmen BR, Gerber C. Analysis of a retrieved Delta III total shoulder prosthesis. J Bone Joint Surg Br 2004;86(8):1187–1191
8. Gotterson PR, Nusem I, Pearcy MJ, Crawford RW. Metal debris from bony resection in knee arthroplasty–is it an issue? Acta Orthop 2005;76(4):475–480
9. von Knoch M, Jewison DE, Sibonga JD, et al. The effectiveness of polyethylene versus titanium particles in inducing osteolysis in vivo. J Orthop Res 2004;22(2):237–243
10. Favard L, Lautmann S, Sirveaux F, Oudet D, Kerjean Y, Huquet D. Hemi arthroplasty versus reverse arthroplasty in the treatment of osteoarthritis with massive rotator cuff tear. In: Walch G, Boileau P, Mole D, eds. 2000 Shoulder Prosthesis. Two To Ten Year Follow-Up. Montpellier, France: Sauramps Medical; 2001: 261–268
11. Gagey O, Hue E. Mechanics of the deltoid muscle. A new approach. Clin Orthop Relat Res 2000;375:250–257
12. Halder AM, Itoi E, An KN. Anatomy and biomechanics of the shoulder. Orthop Clin North Am 2000;31(2):159–176
13. Frankle M, Siegal S, Pupello D, Saleem A, Mighel lM, Vasey M. The Reverse Shoulder Prosthesis for glenohumeral arthritis associated with severe rotator cuff deficiency. A minimum two-year follow-up study of sixty patients. J Bone Joint Surg Am 2005;87(8):1697–1705
14. Copeland S. The continuing development of shoulder replacement: "reaching the surface. J Bone Joint Surg Am 2006;88(4):900–905
15. Jasty M, Bragdon C, Burke D, O'Connor D, Lowenstein J, Harris WH. In vivo skeletal responses to porous-surfaced implants subjected to small induced motions. J Bone Joint Surg Am 1997; 79(5):707–714
16. Franklin JL, Barrett WP, Jackins SE, Matsen FA III. Glenoid loosening in total shoulder arthroplasty. Association with rotator cuff deficiency. J Arthroplasty 1988;3(1):39–46
17. Gutiérrez S, Lott J, Frankle MA, Lee W. Screw failure in a Reverse Shoulder Prosthesis. Paper presented at: 2nd International Symposium: Treatment Of Complex Shoulder Problems; January 13–15, 2005; Tampa, FL
18. Harman M, Frankle M, Vasey M, Banks S. Initial glenoid component fixation in "reverse" total shoulder arthroplasty: a biomechanical evaluation. J Shoulder Elbow Surg 2005a; 14(1, Suppl S)162S–167S
19. Gutiérrez S, Greiwe RM, Frankle MA, Siegal SE, Lee WE II. Biomechanical comparison of component position and hardware failure in the Reverse Shoulder Prosthesis. J Shoulder Elbow Surg, 2007 May-June; 16(3 Suppl):S9–S12
20. Buckwalter JA, Einhorn TA, Simon SR, eds. Orthopaedic Basic Science: Biology and Biomechanics of the Musculoskeletal System (2nd ed). Rosemont, IL: American Academy of Orthopaedic Surgeons, 2000
21. Li K, Saigal S, Frankle M. Effect of base-plate inclination on the fixation of the Reverse Shoulder Prosthesis. Paper presented at: 2nd International Symposium: Treatment of Complex Shoulder Problems; January 13–15, 2005; Tampa, FL
22. Frankle M, Pupello D, Levy J, Gutiérrez S. Component positioning and hardware failure in the Reverse Shoulder Prosthesis. Poster presented at: American Academy of Orthopaedic Surgeons Annual Meeting; March 22–26, 2006; Chicago, IL
23. Harman MK, Frankle M, Banks SA. In-vitro biomechanical analysis of different RSP sizes. Paper presented at: 2nd International Symposium: Treatment of Complex Shoulder Problems; January 13–15, 2005; Tampa, FL
24. Li K, Saigal S, Frankle M. Effect of component size and lateral offset on the fixation of the Reverse Shoulder Prosthesis. Paper presented at: 2nd International Symposium: Treatment Of Complex Shoulder Problems; January 13–15, 2005; Tampa, FL
25. Explanation, copyright 2001–2006. In: TimeWeb. Retrieved June 22, 2006, from <http://www.bized.ac.uk/timeweb/crunching/crunch_relate_expl.htm>
26. Trojani C, Chuinard C. Problems related to the humerus: (intraoperative and postoperative humeral fractures, loosening, unscrewing, subsidence, rotation). Poster presented at: Nice Shoulder Course 2006: Arthroscopy & Arthroplasty Current Concepts. Palais de la Méditerranée; June 3, 2006; Nice, France
27. Nové-Josserand L. Prosthetic instability: clinical presentation (early, late), type of reduction, unique or recurrent, causes, etiologies, treatments, results. Poster presented at: Nice Shoulder Course 2006: Arthroscopy & Arthroplasty Current Concepts. Palais de la Méditerranée; June 3, 2006; Nice, France
28. De Wilde LF, Van Ovost E, Uyttendaele D, Verdonk R. Results of an inverted shoulder prosthesis after resection for tumor of the proximal humerus. Rev Chir Orthop Reparatrice Appar Mot 2002; 88(4):373–378
29. Anglin C, Wyss UP, Pichora DR. Shoulder prosthesis subluxation: theory and experiment. J Shoulder Elbow Surg 2000;9(2):104–114
30. Seebauer L, Walter W, Key IW. Reverse total shoulder arthroplasty for the treatment of defect arthropathy. Oper Orthop Traumatol 2005;17(1):1–24

31. Nyffeler RW, Werner CM, Gerber C. Biomechanical relevance of glenoid component positioning in the reverse Delta III total shoulder prosthesis. J Shoulder Elbow Surg 2005;14(5):524–528

32. de Leest O, Rozing PM, Rozendaal LA, van der Helm FC. Influence of glenohumeral prosthesis geometry and placement on shoulder muscle forces. Clin Orthop Relat Res 1996;330:222–233

33. Frankle M, Virani N, Pupello D, Levy J. Range specific strength following Reverse Shoulder Prosthesis. Poster presented at: 20th Congress for the European Society for Surgery of the Shoulder and the Elbow; September 20–23, 2006; Athens, Greece

34. Broström LA, Wallensten R, Olsson E, Anderson D. The Kessel prosthesis in total shoulder arthroplasty. A five-year experience. Clin Orthop Relat Res 1992;277:155–160

35. Fenlin JM Jr. Total glenohumeral joint replacement. Orthop Clin North Am 1975;6(2):565–583

36. Gerard Y, Leblanc JP, Rousseau B. A complete shoulder prosthesis. Chirurgie 1973;99(9):655–663

37. Kolbel R, Friedebold G. Shoulder joint replacement. Arch Orthop Unfallchir 1973;76(1):31–39

38. Neer CS II, Craig EV, Fukuda H. Cuff-tear arthropathy. J Bone Joint Surg Am 1983;65(9):1232–1244

39. Valenti P, Boutens D, Nerot C., et al. Delta 3 reversed prosthesis for osteoarthritis with massive rotator cuff tear: long term results (>5 years) In: Walch G, Boileau P, Mole D, eds. 2000 Shoulder Prosthesis. Two To Ten Year Follow-Up. Montpellier, France: Sauramps Medical; 2001: 253–259

40. Vanhove B, Beugnies A. Grammont's reverse shoulder prosthesis for rotator cuff arthropathy. A retrospective study of 32 cases. Acta Orthop Belg 2004;70(3):219–225

41. Karduna AR, Williams GR, Williams JL, Iannotti JP. Glenohumeral joint translations before and after total shoulder arthroplasty. A study in cadavera. J Bone Joint Surg Am 1997a;79(8):1166–1174

42. Karduna AR, Williams GR, Williams JL, Iannotti JP. Joint stability after total shoulder arthroplasty in a cadaver model. J Shoulder Elbow Surg 1997b;6(6):506–511

43. Oosterom R, Herder JL, van der Helm FC, Swieszkowski W, Bersee HE. Translational stiffness of the replaced shoulder joint. J Biomech 2003;36(12):1897–1907

44. Weldon EJ III, Scarlat MM, Lee SB, Matsen FA III. Intrinsic stability of unused and retrieved polyethylene glenoid components. J Shoulder Elbow Surg 2001;10(5):474–481

45. Levy J, Frankle M, Mighell M, Pupello D. Use of the reverse shoulder prosthesis for the treatment of failed hemiarthroplasty in patients with glenohumeral arthritis and rotator cuff deficiency. J Bone Joint Surg Br 2007 Feb;89(2):189–95.

46. Guery J, Favard L, Sirveaux F, Oudet D, Mole D, Walch G. Reverse total shoulder arthroplasty. Survivorship analysis of eighty replacements followed for five to ten years. J Bone Joint Surg Am 2006 Aug;88(8):1742–7

47. Wall B, Nové-Josserand L, O'Connor DP, Edwards TB, Walch G. Reverse total shoulder arthroplasty: a review of results according to etiology. J Bone Joint Surg Am 2007 Jul;89(7):1476–85

48. De Wilde LF, Plasschaert FS, Audenaert EA, Verdonk RC. Functional recovery after a reverse prosthesis for reconstruction of the proximal humerus in tumor surgery. Clin Orthop Relat Res 2005 Jan;(430):156–62

49. Paladini P, Collu A, Campi E, Porcellini G. The inverse prosthesis as a revision prosthesis in failures of shoulder hemiarthroplasty. Chir Organi Mov 2005 Jan-Mar;90(1):11–21

50. Seitz WH. The Delta Experience: Does it Fly? Semin Arthro 268–273 2005 Elsevier Inc.

51. De Wilde L, Sys G, Julien Y, Van Ovost E, Poffyn B, Trouilloud P. The reversed Delta shoulder prosthesis in reconstruction of the proximal humerus after tumour resection. Acta Orthop Belg 2003 Dec;69(6):495–500.

52. Katzer A, Sickelmann F, Seemann K, Loehr JF. Two-year results after exchange shoulder arthroplasty using inverse implants. Orthopedics. 2004 Nov;27(11):1165–7

53. Woodruff MJ, Cohen AP, Bradley JG. Arthroplasty of the shoulder in rheumatoid arthritis with rotator cuff dysfunction. Int Orthop 2003;27(1):7–10. Epub 2002 Oct 23

54. Boulahia A, Edwards TB, Walch G, Baratta RV. Early results of a reverse design prosthesis in the treatment of arthritis of the shoulder in elderly patients with a large rotator cuff tear. Orthopedics 2002 Feb;25(2):129–33.

55. Rittmeister M, Kerschbaumer F. Grammont reverse total shoulder arthroplasty in patients with rheumatoid arthritis and nonreconstructible rotator cuff lesions. J Shoulder Elbow Surg 2001 Jan-Feb;10(1):17–22

56. De Wilde L, Mombert M, Van Petegem P, Verdonk R. Revision of shoulder replacement with a reversed shoulder prosthesis (Delta III): report of five cases Acta Orthop Belg. 2001 Oct;67(4):348–53

57. Jacobs R, Debeer P, De Smet L. Treatment of rotator cuff arthropathy with a reversed Delta shoulder prosthesis. Acta Orthop Belg 2001 Oct;67(4):344–7

58. E Baulot, E Garron, and PM Grammont Grammont prosthesis in humeral head osteonecrosis. Indications—results, Acta Orthop Belg 1999, Vol. 65:.109–115

59. Baulot E, Chabernaud D, Grammont PM. Results of Grammont's inverted prosthesis in omarthritis associated with major cuff destruction. Apropos of 16 cases Acta Orthop Belg 1995;61 (Suppl 1):112–9

60. Grammont PM, Baulot E. Delta shoulder prosthesis for rotator cuff rupture. Orthopedics 1993 Jan;16(1):65–8

61. Gutiérrez S, Frankle MA, Levy JC, Cuff D, Keller TS, Pupello DR, Lee III WEE. Evaluation of abduction range of motion and avoidance of inferior scapular impingement associated with reverse shoulder implants. J Shoulder Elbow Surg. In press.

9 Rationale and Biomechanics of the Reversed Shoulder Prosthesis: The French Experience

Pascal Boileau and Christopher Chuinard

The Problem

Treatment of the cuff-deficient shoulder has been a vexing problem for many years. Although the rotator cuff provides control of overhead rotation of the humerus and internal and external rotation (ER) of the arm, its main function is to stabilize the humeral head in the confines of the glenoid, thereby creating a stable fulcrum around which the deltoid can act, providing forward flexion of the humerus.

When the rotator cuff is torn, the dynamic balance of the shoulder can be lost; however, not every advanced cuff tear (CT) leads to loss of forward flexion beyond 90 degrees (i.e., pseudoparalysis). In fact, some patients can present with complete tears of the posterior cuff, but maintain forward flexion if there is a balance between internal and external rotatory forces. An intact coracoacromial arch can provide a stable articulation allowing the deltoid to work when there is a balance between the subscapularis and teres minor.

If the dynamic balance of the joint is lost and arthropathy ensues, what options are available? Constrained arthroplasty seemed to provide great promise for restoration of function because the humerus could be stabilized, allowing the deltoid to work. Completely constrained ball and socket designs, introduced in the 1970s, were adapted from hip prostheses (Bickel, Macnab-English, Stanmore, Michael-Reese, Post).[1,8] Subsequently, several prostheses were introduced based on a reverse ball-and-socket design (Fenlin, Gerard, Kessel, Kölbel, Liverpool, Neer, and Avery II).[2,33] To achieve appropriate resting length and tension on the deltoid, the original reverse ball and socket designs lateralized the humeral component; concomitantly, the center of rotation was lateralized. In fact, the instant center of rotation was lateralized outside of the scapula, creating a lever arm between the center of rotation and the bone/implant interface. Because of the vectors involved with humeral movement below 90 degrees (i.e., the initiation of abduction or humeral flexion), both torque and sheer between the implant and the bone were created, resulting in loosening (**Fig. 9–1**).

Moreover, the constraint between the humeral and the glenoid components meant that all of the forces were transmitted to the glenoscapular interface. The failures and poor results led to abandonment of both reverse architecture and constrained designs. Experience with uncon-

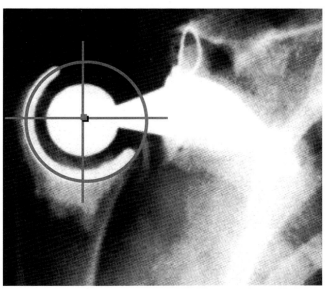

Figure 9–1 Previous reverse ball and socket prostheses tended to fail because their design resulted in excessive torque or shear forces on the glenoid component (notice the small head and neck placing the center of rotation outside the scapula).

strained total shoulder arthroplasty for the cuff-deficient shoulder was also unsatisfying as the "rocking-horse" effect led to early failure, and hemiarthroplasty became the recommended treatment.[3,4] Bipolar arthroplasty gained a brief following, and has remained the procedure of choice for a select few.[5,6-19]

The Vision

Dissatisfied with the results of standard architecture arthroplasty for the cuff-deficient shoulder, Professor Paul Grammont, a French orthopedic surgeon, designed a semi-constrained reverse prosthesis based on different, but sound, biomechanical principles. To replicate the stability of the intact cuff, a semiconstrained design was chosen to give the deltoid a stable fulcrum; to give mechanical advantage to the deltoid, he increased its resting length and recruited the posterior deltoid.

Prior to Grammont, constrained shoulder prostheses tended to fail because their design resulted in excessive torque and shear forces at the glenoid component–bone interface. Furthermore, although they usually allowed some active elevation, this was, in most cases, less than 90 degrees and, primarily, scapulothoracic motion. Prosthetic instability was also a concern. Many never went beyond the experimental stage, and most are no longer commercially available.

Grammont recognized that the lateral center of rotation found in previous designs created a large lever arm between the "ball" and its bone interface. By medializing the center of rotation (so that it actually lies at the glenoid bone–prosthesis interface), Grammont reduced the torque on the glenoid component. Furthermore, with initiation of abduction, the vector changed from parallel to the component/scapula interface (i.e., shear) to perpendicular to the glenoid component (i.e., compression), theoretically increasing stability of the construct when it is most vulnerable (**Fig. 9–2**).

To power the "engine" of this new design, the deltoid, Grammont sought to maximize the resting tension on the deltoid while involving more of both the anterior and the posterior fibers. To effect the changes in the deltoid, a combined inferiorization and medialization of the humerus relative to the acromion increases deltoid tension and resting length, recruiting more anterior and posterior deltoid fibers and improving the force vectors (**Fig. 9–3**).

The realization of these principles involved two major technological innovations: (1) on the glenoid side, use of a large ball (36 or 42 mm in diameter) with no neck; (2) on the humeral side, a small cup inclined to a non-anatomic humeral inclination of 155 degrees with conforming—but not fully constrained—articular surfaces. Both the large glenoid hemisphere and the small and conforming humeral cup optimize the range of movement, minimize impingement between the components, and improve stability.

The first model of reverse prosthesis, designed by Paul Grammont in 1985, had only two components (**Fig. 9–4**). The glenoid component was either a metallic or a ceramic ball, initially two thirds of a sphere and 42 mm in diameter. It was designed to fit over the glenoid like a glove and was fixed with cement. The humeral component was a cemented polyethylene socket. Its concave surface was one third of a sphere, and its stem was trumpet-shaped for cementing into the humeral medullary canal. A bell saw was used to prepare the glenoid, and two broaches were used to prepare the different parts of the humerus—one for the epiphysis and one for the diaphysis.

The preliminary results published (in French) in 1987 showed eight cases: three post-radiotherapy necrosis cases, one inflammatory osteoarthritis case, and four revisions of failed prostheses.[9] The mean patient age was 70 years, and the cuff was absent or destroyed in all cases. Mean follow-up was only 6 months. A transacromial approach (with osteotomy of the lateral acromion) was used in all but one case. Revision osteosynthesis of an acromial nonunion was required in three cases. All shoulders were pain-free, but mobility was variable. In three cases, active anterior elevation was 100 to 130 degrees, but in the other three cases, it was less than 60 degrees.

The Realization

Unsatisfied with these results, Grammont made further modifications, arriving at the current design. Because he had several failures with the cemented glenoid component, he decided to change the glenoid to an uncemented system: a glenoid component fixed with a press-fit central peg supported by screws of divergent direction that counteract the initial shearing forces.[2,9] He also changed the ra-

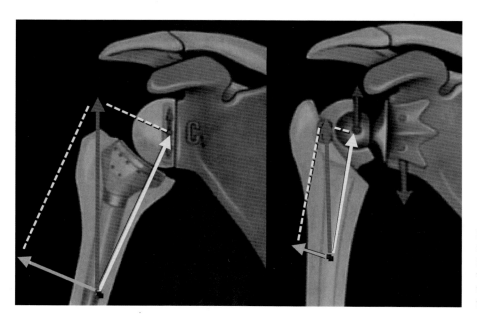

Figure 9–2 By placing the center of rotation medial, torsion and shear at the bone–glenoid interface are reduced; furthermore, with the adduction, the force vector goes from parallel to the articular surface (shear) to perpendicular (compression).

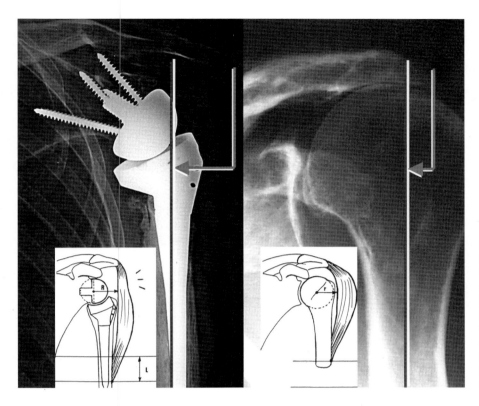

Figure 9–3 (A,B) The increased force of the deltoid is gained from both the medialization of the center of rotation, which recruits more deltoid fibers, and the lowering of the humerus, which tensions the deltoid. (A) L = increased length. The figure shows a shoulder with a reverse prosthesis and compares the center of rotation and humeral position to a native glenohumeral joint (B). There is an obvious increase in acromiohumeral distance and an overall lengthening of the humerus.

dius of the articular surface from two thirds of a sphere to half of a sphere to place the center of rotation directly in contact with the glenoid surface, decreasing lateral offset

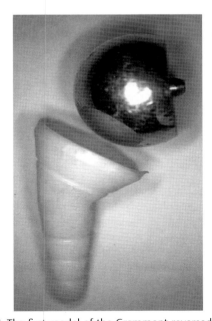

Figure 9–4 The first model of the Grammont reversed prosthesis, designed in 1985, had only two components: the humeral component was all polyethylene and trumpet shaped; the glenoid component was a metallic or ceramic ball, initially $^2/_3$ of a sphere and 42 mm in diameter. It was designed to fit over the glenoid like a glove and was affixed with cement.

at the glenohumeral articulation, thus decreasing shearing forces. Grammont named this reverse prosthesis "Delta," as the concept was based solely on the deltoid for both function and stability.

The second model, the Delta III reverse prosthesis (DePuy Orthopaedics, Inc., Warsaw, Indiana), became available in 1991 and is still in use today. The glenoid is uncemented, and either cemented or uncemented options are available for the humerus. The Delta III has five parts: the glenoid base plate (metaglenoid), the glenosphere, the polyethylene humeral cup, the humeral neck, and the humeral stem (**Fig. 9–5**).

The glenoid component (metaglene) is a 29-mm disk, with a rough surface and hydroxyapatite coating. Initial fixation is ensured by a 29-mm-long central peg and four peripheral, divergent screws (3.5 or 4.5 mm in diameter). The aim is to place one screw in the base of the coracoid and one screw into the inferior scapular pillar for maximum hold. The pyramidal, divergent assembly of the screws has been designed precisely to counteract the shearing forces during initial abduction.

The glenosphere is a cobalt-chrome sphere, available in two diameters: 36 and 42 mm, with a 19-mm offset. Initially, the fixation of the sphere on the metaglene was done by use of peripheral threads, but this mechanism had a tendency to unscrew, particularly in right shoulders. In 1996, glenosphere-metaglene fixation was changed to a peripheral Morse taper and reinforced by a central countersunk screw; the design change has almost completely eliminated glenosphere dissociation except in trauma cases.

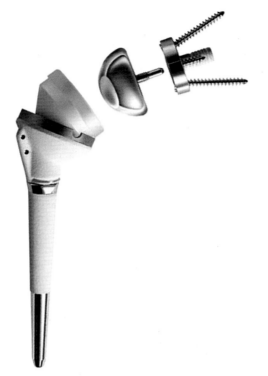

Figure 9–5 The Delta III reversed prosthesis has five parts: the glenoid base plate (metaglenoid), the glenosphere, the polyethylene cup, the humeral neck, and the humeral stem. A lateralized spacer, the rehausser (not pictured), can provide greater deltoid tension if the polyethylene is insufficient. Both a Delta I and a Delta II exist, but they are variations of a conventional arthroplasty that utilize the same humeral stem.

The humeral stem is conical, and its surface is either polished or hydroxyapatite-coated for cemented or uncemented fixation, respectively. It is available in three lengths: 100 mm for the standard prosthesis and 150 and 180 mm for the revision prosthesis.

The humeral neck is screwed onto the humeral stem. It has a fin to control rotation, and there are holes to allow tuberosity osteosynthesis. Like the stem, it is available with a polished or a hydroxyapatite-coated surface. Three sizes are available: 36–1 and 36–2 for a 36-mm-diameter cup and 42–2 for a 42-mm-diameter cup. Initial unscrewing between the neck and the stem resulted in the placement of a polyethylene bushing between these components.

The humeral cup is made of polyethylene and has two diameters conforming to the 36- and 42-mm glenospheres. It is 6 mm thick and press-fitted onto the humeral neck component. A 9-mm metallic extension may be screwed onto the neck to increase the humeral offset. The humeral cup is also available in a more constrained form with a deeper cup.

The Delta I and II prostheses are "standard" unconstrained versions of the Delta III prosthesis. All three prostheses share the same stem and humeral neck. The Delta I is a hemiarthroplasty, which is easily converted from a Delta III by fixing a metal head onto the humeral neck, whereas the Delta II is a total shoulder prosthesis with a polyethylene glenoid component in place of the glenosphere.

A further evolution of Grammont's designs occurred under the direction of Dr. Gilles Walch and Prof. Pascal Boileau. The Aequalis reverse prosthesis, available since 2002, follows the Grammont design, but incorporates prosthetic changes designed to enhance both the ease of implantation and survivability: improved instrumentation, variable angle locking screws, and an array of polyethylene thicknesses.

The baseplate maintains the titanium HA design, but adds the ability to vary the direction of the locking screws up to 30 degrees superiorly for the upper screw and 30 degrees inferiorly for the lower screw; furthermore, they both can be angled ±15 degrees in the anteroposterior (AP) direction.

For the humeral component, a polyethylene bushing was added between the neck and the stem to minimize the risk of disassembly. The cemented stem is rough-finished cobalt chromium with scalloping to increase rotational stability; the noncemented stem is titanium with HA coating. There are four stem lengths available—100 mm, 150 mm, 180 mm, and 210 mm. There are three polyethylene sizes available: 6 mm, 9 mm, and 12 mm, plus an additional 9-mm titanium spacer. A humeral head adaptor to accommodate an Aequalis standard head is available should the prosthesis need to be converted to a hemiarthroplasty.

The Deltoid and Grammont's Design

This design confers mobility, increased deltoid torque, and stability, while minimizing the unfavorable glenoid stresses, which led to the failure of previous reverse prostheses. According to Grammont, the middle deltoid is most important for abduction. This is particularly true in a normal shoulder where parts of the anterior and posterior deltoid are at the level of, or even medial to the center of rotation;[8] therefore, they either contribute very little to abduction or, in the case of the more medial fibers, may even be adductors. However, in patients with a reverse prosthesis, the medialized center of rotation may allow some of these fibers to become more effective abductors, thus augmenting the role of the anterior and posterior deltoid and further increasing the force of the deltoid overall (**Fig. 9–6**).

To effect the necessary changes to the deltoid, it must be tensioned despite the medialization of the humerus. Unfortunately, intraoperative determination of deltoid tension is difficult and guided mostly by surgical experience; reduction should be as tight as possible, but allow for full adduction. We also have found that the conjoint tendon, exposed during a deltopectoral approach, should feel taut after reduction with the arm at the side and the elbow extended.

Biomechanics of the Grammont Design

Active elevation is restored by the fixed center of rotation, the congruent joint surfaces, and the increased deltoid

Table 9–2   Groups and Treatment for Cuff Tear Arthropathy

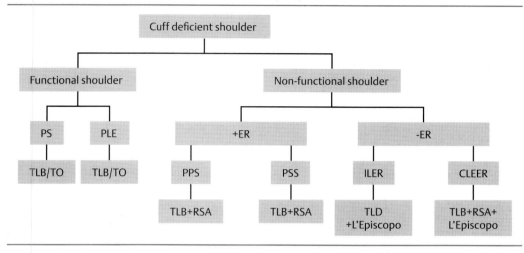

Abbreviations: PS, pseudoparalyzed; PLE, painful loss of elevation; TLB/TO, tenodesis of the long head of biceps/tenotomy of biceps; ER, external rotation; PSS, painful stiff shoulder; ILER, isolated loss of external rotation; CLEER, combined loss of elevation and external rotation; RSA, reverse shoulder arthroplasty.

Group 1 – Painful Shoulder   Patients only complain of pain; they have normal or near normal active elevation and ER. They may have lost the last 20 or 30 degrees of *passive* elevation because of entrapment of a hypertrophic biceps tendon (hourglass biceps).[42] The acromiohumeral distance (AHD) may be normal, but is usually decreased (<7 mm) and there is minimal to no osteoarthritis (OA) or necrosis (Hamada and Fukuda stages 1, 2, or 3). The infraspinatus, if present, has fatty infiltration (Goutallier stage 3 or 4), but the teres minor is normal or hypertrophic. These patients are best treated with an arthroscopic biceps tenotomy or tenodesis. A partial cuff repair may be associated. An acromioplasty is not recommended, but can be performed if the AHD is >7 mm.

Group 2 – Painful Loss of Elevation   Patients complain of both pain and loss of active elevation; they have normal or near normal active ER. Passive elevation is usually normal, and the patients can maintain elevation above 90 degrees if the arm is assisted to this position (the descent test). The loss of active elevation is linked to the severity of the pain and can be improved with a lidocaine injection. Again, the AHD is usually decreased (<7 mm) but there is little or no OA or necrosis (Hamada and Fukuda stages 1, 2, or 3). The infraspinatus is fatty infiltrated (Goutallier stage 3 or 4) or torn, but the teres minor is normal or hypertrophic. These patients are also best treated with an arthroscopic biceps tenotomy or tenodesis. A partial cuff repair may be associated. An acromioplasty is not recommended, but can be performed if the AHD is >7 mm.

Group 3 – Pseudoparalyzed Shoulder   Patients complain of loss of active elevation, but maintain normal

passive elevation; they have normal or near normal active ER. There is anterosuperior escape of the humeral head with attempted elevation of the arm (shrug). The acromiohumeral is usually decreased (<7 mm). There may be OA or necrosis (Hamada and Fukuda stage 3 or 4); however, some patients have a pseudoparalyzed shoulder and no OA (Hamada stage 1, 2, 3). The infraspinatus, if present, is fatty infiltrated (Goutallier stage 3 or 4), but the teres minor is normal or hypertrophic. The subscapularis is often torn or fatty infiltrated, and the long head of the biceps is often dislocated. These patients are best treated with a reverse prosthesis and a biceps tenotomy or tenodesis.

Group 4 – Painful Stiff Shoulder   Patients complain of painful loss of active and passive elevation; they also have limited active and passive ER (internal contracture). The AHD is usually decreased (<7 mm). There is OA or necrosis (Hamada and Fukuda stage 3 or 4). The infraspinatus may be fatty infiltrated or torn. These patients are best treated with a reverse prosthesis and a biceps tenotomy or tenodesis.

Group 5 – Isolated Loss of ER   Patients complain of isolated loss of active ER, but active elevation is normal or near normal. Pain is usually present, but may resolve if there is a spontaneous rupture of the biceps. The impairment of active ER is demonstrated by the presence of the hornblower sign, the drop sign, and the ER lag sign (ERLS).[22,43] The acromiohumeral is usually decreased (<7 mm), but there is little to no OA or necrosis (Hamada stage 1, 2, 3). Both the infraspinatus and teres minor are torn or completely fatty infiltrated (Goutallier stage 3 or 4). The subscapularis is normal or partially torn. These patients are best treated with a latissimus dorsi and teres major transfer and a biceps tenotomy or tenodesis.

Group 6 – Combined Loss of Elevation and External Rotation   Patients complain of combined loss of active elevation and active ER. They have normal passive elevation and rotation. There is anterosuperior escape of the humeral head with attempted elevation of the arm (shrug). The acromiohumeral is usually decreased (<7 mm). There may be OA or necrosis (Hamada and Fukuda stage 3 or 4), but some patients have a combined loss of elevation and ER without OA (Hamada stage 1, 2, 3). The infraspinatus and teres minor are both completely fatty infiltrated (Goutallier stage 3 or 4). The subscapularis is

often torn or fatty infiltrated and the long head of the biceps is pathologic. These patients are best treated with a reverse prosthesis, biceps tenotomy, or tenodesis and an associated latissimus dorsi and teres major transfer.

Unlike previous reverse ball and socket designs, the Grammont reverse prosthesis creates a new biomechanical environment for the deltoid muscle, replicating the stabilizing effect of the rotator cuff muscles, providing a stable fulcrum for the deltoid, and minimizing shearing forces on the glenoid component. His design has obviated early failure due to glenoid loosening and should be considered a great advancement in the field of shoulder arthroplasty. Clinical follow-up remains short to medium-term at present, but the Grammont reverse prosthesis shows promise where its predecessors have failed.

References

1. Coughlin MJ, Morris JM, West WF. The semiconstrained total shoulder arthroplasty. J Bone Joint Surg Am 1979;61:574–581
2. Grammont PM, Baulot E. Delta shoulder prosthesis for rotator cuff rupture. Orthopedics. 1993;16:65–68
3. Kapandjil A. The shoulder. Clin Rheum Dis 1982;8:595–616
4. Bayley JIL, Kessel L. The Kessel total shoulder replacement. In: Bayley J, Kessel L, eds. Shoulder Surgery. New York, NY: Springer; 1982
5. Field LD, Dines DM, Zabinski SJ, Warren RF. Hemiarthroplasty of the shoulder for rotator cuff arthropathy. J Shoulder Elbow Surg 1997;6:18–23
6. Pollock RG, Deliz ED, McIlveen SJ, Flatow EL, Bigliani LU. Prosthetic replacement in rotator cuff deficient shoulders. J Shoulder Elbow Surg 1992;1:173–186
7. Worland RL, Jessup DE, Arredondo J, Warburton KJ. Bipolar shoulder arthoplasty for rotator cuff arthropathy. J Shoulder Elbow Surg 1997;6:512–515
8. Sanchez-Sotelo J, Cofield RH, Rowland CM. Shoulder hemiarthroplasty for glenohumeral arthritis associated with severe rotator cuff deficiency. J Bone Joint Surg Am 2001;83:1814–1822
9. Grammont P, Trouilloud P, Laffay JP, Deries X. Etude et réalisation d'une nouvelle prothèse d'épaule. Rhumatologie 1987;39:17–22
10. Grammont PM, Baulot E, Chabernaud D. Résultats des 16 premiers cas d'arthroplastie totale d'épaule inversée sans ciment pour des omarthroses avec grande rupture de coiffe. Rev Chir Orthop Reparatrice Appar Mot 1996;82(suppl I):169
11. Jacobs R, DeBeer P, De Smet L. Treatment of rotator cuff arthropathy with reversed delta shoulder prosthesis. Acta Orthop Belg 2001;67:344–347
12. Fick R. Handbuch der Anatomie und Mekanik Gelenke. Iéna, Germany: Gustave Fischer; 1911
13. Strasser H. Lehrbuch der Muskel und Gelenkmechanik. Berlin, Germany: J. Springer; 1917
14. DeWilde L, Audenaert E, Barbaix E, Audenaert A, Soudan K. Consequences of deltoid muscle elongation on deltoid muscle performance: a computerized study. Clin Biomech (Bristol, Avon) 2002;17:499–505
15. Crowninshield RD, Maloney WJ, Wentz DH, Humphrey SM, Blanchard CR. Biomechanics of large femoral heads: what they do and don't do. Clin Orthop Relat Res 2004;429:102–107
16. Rittmeister M, Kersch Baumer F. Grammont reverse total shoulder arthroplasty in patients with rheumatoid arthritis and non-reconstructible rotator cuff lesions. J Shoulder Elbow Surg 2001;10:17–22
17. Sirveaux F, Favard L, Oudet D, Huguet D, Lautman S. Grammont inverted total shoulder arthroplasty in the treatment of glenohumeral osteoarthritis with massive and non repairable cuff rupture. In: Walch G, Boileau P, Molé D, eds. 2000 Shoulder Prosthesis... Two To Ten Year Follow-Up. Montpellier, France: Sauramps Medical; 2001: 247–252
18. Edwards TB, Boulahia A, Kempf JF, Boileau P, Nemoz C, Walch G. The influence of the rotator cuff on the results of shoulder arthroplasty for primary osteoarthritis: results of a multicenter study. J Bone Joint Surg Am 2002;84:2240–2248
19. Valenti P, Boutens D, Nerot C. Delta 3 reversed prosthesis for arthritis with massive rotator cuff tear: long term results (> 5 years). In: Walch G, Boileau P, Molé D, eds. 2000 Shoulder Prosthesis... Two To Ten Year Follow-Up. Montpellier, France: Sauramps Medical; 2001:253–259
20. Boileau P, Watkinson DJ, Hatzidakis A, Balg F. The Grammont reverse prosthesis: Design, rationale and biomechanics. J Shoulder Elbow Surg 2005;14(Supp. I):147S–161S
21. Nyffeler RW, Werner CM, Gerber C. Biomechanical relevance of glenoid component positioning in the reversed Delta III total shoulder prosthesis. J Shoulder Elbow Surg 2005;14:524–528
22. Walch G, Boulahia A, Calderone S, Robinson AHN. The dropping and hornblower's signs in evaluation of rotator cuff tears. J Bone Joint Surg Br 1998;80:624–628
23. Constant CR, Murley AHG. A clinical method of functional assessment of the shoulder. Clin Orthop Relat Res 1987;214:160–164
24. DeButtet A, Bouchon Y, Capon D, Delfosse J. Grammont shoulder arthroplasty for osteoarthritis with massive rotator cuff tears: report of 71 cases. J Shoulder Elbow Surg 1997;6:197
25. Nove-Josserend L, Walch G, Wall B. Instability of the reverse prosthesis. In: Walch G, Boileau P, Molé D, Favard L, Lévigne C, Sirveaux F, eds. Reverse Shoulder Arthroplasty. Montpellier, France: Sauramps Medical; 2006:247–260
26. Chuinard C, Trojani C, Brassart N, Boileau P. Humeral problems in reverse total shoulder arthroplasty. In: Walch G, Boileau P, Molé D, Favard L, Lévigne C, Sirveaux F, eds. Reverse Shoulder Arthroplasty. Montpellier, France: Sauramps Medical; 2006:275–288
27. DeWilde L, Mombert M, Vanpetegem P, Verdonk R. Revision of shoulder replacement with a reversed shoulder prosthesis (Delta III). Report of five cases. Acta Orthop Belg 2001;67:348–353
28. Sirveaux F, Favard L, Oudet D, Huguet D, Walch G, Mole D. Grammont inverted total shoulder arthroplasty in the treatment of glenohumeral osteoarthritis with massive rupture of the cuff. Re-

sults of a multicentre study of 80 shoulders. J Bone Joint Surg Br 2004;86:388–395

29. Boulahia A, Edwards TB, Walch G, Baratta RV. Early results of a reverse design prosthesis in the treatment of arthritis of the shoulder in elderly patients with a large rotator cuff tear. Orthopedics 2002;25:129–133

30. Broström LÅ, Wallenstein R, Olsson E, Anderson D. The Kessel prosthesis in total shoulder arthroplasty. A five-year experience. Clin Orthop Relat Res 1992;277:155–160

31. DeWilde LF, Van Ovost E, Uyttendaele D, Verdonk R. Results of an inverted shoulder prosthesis after resection for tumor of the proximal humerus. Rev Chir Orthop Reparatrice Appar Mot 2002;88:373–378

32. Favard L, Lautmann S, Sirveaux F, Oudet D, Kerjean Y, Huguet D. Hemi arthroplasty versus reverse arthroplasty in the treatment of osteoarthritis with massive rotator cuff tear. In: Walch G, Boileau P, Molé D, eds. 2000 Shoulder Prosthesis... Two To Ten Year Follow-Up. Montpellier, France: Sauramps Medical; 2001: 261–268

33. Werner CM, Steinmann PA, Gilbart M, Gerber C. Treatment of painful pseudoparesis due to irreparable rotator cuff dysfunction with the Delta III reverse-ball-and-socket total shoulder prosthesis. J Bone Joint Surg Am 2005;87:1476–1486

34. Nyffeler RW, Werner CM, Simmen BR, Gerber C. Analysis of a retrieved Delta III total shoulder prosthesis. J Bone Joint Surg Br 2004;86:1187–1191

35. Levigne C, Boileau P, Favard L, et al. Scapular notching in reverse shoulder arthroplasty. In: Walch G, Boileau P, Molé D, Favard L, Lévigne C, Sirveaux F, eds. Reverse Shoulder Arthroplasty. Montpellier, France: Sauramps Medical; 2006:353–372

36. Coste J, Reig S, Trojani C, Berg M, Walch G, Boileau P. The management of infection in arthroplasty of the shoulder. J Bone Joint Surg Br 2004;86:65–69

37. Jacquot N, Chuinard C, Boileau P. Results of deep infection after shoulder arthroplasty. In: Walch G, Boileau P, Molé D, Favard L, Lévigne C, Sirveaux F, eds. Reverse Shoulder Arthroplasty. Montpellier, France: Sauramps Medical; 2006:303–314

38. Baulot E, Chabernaud D, Grammont P. Résultats de la prothèse inversée de Grammont pour les omarthroses associées à de grandes destructions de la coiffe. A propos de 16 cas. Acta Orthop Belg 1995;61(suppl. I):112–119

39. Boileau P, Trojani C, Chuinard C, Lehuec JC, Walch G. Proximal humerus fracture sequelae: impact of a new radiographic classification on arthroplasty. Clin Orthop Relat Res 2006;442:121–130

40. Frankle M. Reverse shoulder prosthesis can successfully treat patients that failed due to recurrent instability. Paper presented at: 9th International Congress on Surgery of the Shoulder (ICS); May 2–5, 2004Washington, DC

41. Hamada K, Fukuda H. Roentgenographic findings in massive rotator cuff tears. A long-term observation. Clin Orthop Relat Res 1990;254:92–96

42. Boileau P, Ahrens PM, Hatzidakis AM. Entrapment of the long head of the biceps tendon: the hourglass biceps—a cause of pain and locking of the shoulder. J Shoulder Elbow Surg 2004;13:249–257

43. Hertel R, Ballmer FT, Lambert SM, Gerber C. Lag signs in the diagnosis of rotator cuff rupture. J Shoulder Elbow Surg 1996;5:307–313

44. Lee DH, Niemann KM. Bipolar shoulder arthroplasty. Clin Orthop Relat Res 1994;304:97–107

45. Lettin A, Copeland S, Scales J. The Stanmore total shoulder replacement. J Bone Joint Surg Br 1982;64:47–51

46. Levine WN, Djurasovic M, Glasson JM, et al. Hemiarthroplasty for gleno-humeral osteoarthritis: results correlated to degree of glenoid wear. J Shoulder Elbow Surg 1997;6:449–454

47. McElwain J, English E. The early results of porous coated total shoulder arthroplasty. Clin Orthop Relat Res 1987;218:217–224

48. Post M, Haskell SS, Jablon M. Total shoulder replacement with a constrained prosthesis. J Bone Joint Surg Am 1980;62:327–335

49. Swanson AB, de Groot Swanson G, Sattel AB, Cendo RD, Hynes D, Jar-Ning W. Bipolar implant shoulder arthroplasty. Long-term results. Clin Orthop Relat Res 1989;249:227–247

50. Fenlin JM. Total glenohumeral joint replacement. Orthop Clin North Am 1975;6:565–583

51. Kölbel R, Friedebold G. Stabilization of shoulders with bone and muscle defects using joint replacement implants. In: Bateman J, Welsh P, eds. Shoulder Surgery. St. Louis, MO: The C.V. Mosby Company; 1984:281–293

52. Neer CS, Watson KC, Stanton FJ. Recent experience in total shoulder replacement. J Bone Joint Surg Am 1982;64:319–337

53. Williams GR Jr, Rockwood CA Jr. Hemiarthroplasty in rotator cuff-deficient shoulders. J Shoulder Elbow Surg 1996;5:362–367

54. Wirth MA, Rockwood CA Jr. Current concepts review. Complications of total shoulder arthroplasty. J Bone Joint Surg Am 1996;78:603–616

55. Zuckerman JD, Scott AJ, Gallagher MA. Hemiarthroplasty for cuff tear arthropathy. J Shoulder Elbow Surg 2000;9:169–172

56. Frankle M, Siegal S, Pupello D, Saleem A, Mighell M, Vasey M. The reverse shoulder prosthesis for gleno-humeral arthritis associated with severe rotator cuff deficiency. A minimum two-year follow-up study of sixty patients. J Bone Joint Surg Am 2005;87:1697–1705

10 Treating the Rotator Cuff–Deficient Shoulder: The Lyon, France, Experience

Gilles Walch and Bryan Wall

In 1983, Neer[1] first described cuff tear arthropathy (CTA) as glenohumeral arthritis in the presence of a massive rotator cuff (RC) tear and collapse of the humeral head. It was thought that the massive tear preceded the onset of glenohumeral changes, and that the loss of containment of the articular fluid and loss of motion led to improper cartilage nutrition, which progresses to glenohumeral arthritis. In addition, the altered biomechanics of the shoulder resulted in progressive superior migration of the humeral head, which would eventually erode into the underside of the acromion. The end result of this process was acetabulization of the shoulder with collapse of the humeral head.

Hamada and colleagues[2] stratified the progression of massive cuff tears to CTA into a five-tiered system introduced in 1990. Grade 1 included those patients with massive cuff tears and >6 mm of acromiohumeral distance. Grade 2 indicated an acromiohumeral distance ≤6 mm. Severe erosion, or acetabulization, of the acromion occurred in grade 3. Grade 4 has since been subdivided into grade 4a, glenohumeral joint changes without acetabulization, and grade 4b, glenohumeral joint changes with acetabulization.[3] The onset of humeral head collapse is indicated by grade 5.

Clinical Presentation

The patient with the cuff-deficient shoulder may recall an inciting traumatic event; however, the onset is frequently indolent. Immediately after the acute massive tear, pain and weakness are the most common presenting symptoms. As the pain subsides, patients frequently present with a loss of active motion while maintaining normal passive motion, what has been termed the *pseudoparalytic shoulder.*[4]

Active elevation is limited to that which can be achieved through the scapulothoracic junction and is typically <80 degrees. In addition to the loss of active elevation, the clinical examination will often show weakness or loss of active external rotation (ER). This may occur with the elbow either at the patient's side ("dropping sign") or in 90 degrees of abduction ("hornblower's sign"). Prior to the onset of degenerative changes, patients may regain some active motion, but often remain painful and easily fatigable during prolonged or repetitive activity. In time, many will develop significant nocturnal pain with some degree of stiffness. With the onset of glenohumeral changes, pain and stiffness with loss of passive motion will become the dominant symptoms. At this point, there is significant disability and the functional use of the extremity is negligible.

Massive RC tears or degeneration of the cuff muscle can also be seen in cases of primary glenohumeral arthritis.

Treatment

The sheer number of treatment options available indicates the difficulty this problem presents. Nonoperative treatment is generally reserved for those patients who are Hamada grades 1, 2, or 3, with a normal glenohumeral joint and before the onset of true CTA. Pain and loss of motion will be the most common complaints. Nonoperative modalities can consist of antiinflammatory medications, corticosteroid injections, and activity modification. A physical therapy program focused on stretching is often helpful to regain passive and some active range of motion (ROM).

Arthroscopic treatments that have been recommended for this condition include tuberoplasty, débridement with anterior acromioplasty, and biceps tenotomy. Fenlin et al[5] described arthroscopic tuberoplasty for patients with Hamada grade 2 and 3 changes. The goal of the procedure is to create a congruent acromiohumeral articulation by reshaping the proximal humerus. No concomitant acromioplasty is performed, and the coracoacromial arch is maintained to capture the humeral head during active elevation. Good pain relief and functional restoration were reported, but all patients noted poor ER strength. The procedure is relatively low risk, and no complications were reported. The procedure is contraindicated in the presence of glenohumeral arthritis.

Rockwood and colleagues[6,7] have reported on the results of anterior acromioplasty and cuff débridement in association with an aggressive rehabilitation program for the treatment of massive cuff tears. Patients with a strong anterior deltoid and intact biceps did well with significant improvement in active elevation and pain relief; however, patients with a history of previous attempts at cuff repair showed little improvement.

Walch et al[3] described release of the long head of the biceps. Significant improvement in pain score and activities of daily living were noted; however, radiographic signs of glenohumeral arthritis and humeral head migration continued to progress.

Tendon transfers of the latissimus dorsi and pectoralis major have been used with reasonable success in select patients.[8–12] Gerber et al[9] noted good results in patients undergoing latissimus dorsi transfers so long as the subscapularis remained intact. In a similar report, Jost et al[10] reported good results with pectoralis major transfer for subscapularis deficiency, but results were not as good in the presence of a concomitant irreparable supraspinatus tear.

Arthrodesis has been suggested as an open technique for the treatment of massive cuff tears with and without glenohumeral changes. However, the procedure may not be well tolerated by the older patient.[11-17] The effectiveness of this modality may also be limited by the difficulty of obtaining a solid fusion, with pseudarthrosis rates as high as 20%.[12,13-23] The possibility of bilateral shoulder involvement and relatively poor functional outcomes has led some to abandon this technique. The one place that arthrodesis may still be indicated is for the younger manual laborer who has failed prior attempts at cuff repair.[11]

The results of total shoulder arthroplasty in patients with massive cuff tears and glenohumeral degenerative disease have been poor, secondary to early glenoid loosening.[14] The "rocking horse glenoid," as originally described by Franklin and Matsen, leads to excessive force on the superior edge of the glenoid, secondary to head migration.[15] This eccentric loading compromises the glenoid fixation and results in early loosening.

Hemiarthroplasty with limited-goals rehabilitation has been suggested by numerous authors because it avoids the problem of glenoid loosening completely.[1,16-28] Typically, this results in some alleviation of pain, but incomplete restoration of motion, particularly active anterior elevation. Progressive erosion of the undersurface of the acromion can still occur.

Bipolar hemiarthroplasty is a relatively new treatment modality. In theory, the bipolar head design allows better elevation as the head stabilizes the humerus for the deltoid to pull against. Functional results reported using this method have been disappointing and have not led to a dramatic improvement in results when compared with hemiarthroplasty.[16-31]

Reverse total shoulder arthroplasty initially had poor results due to early glenoid loosening.[17,18-39] Grammont reintroduced the concept in the early 1990s, using an improved prosthetic design.[19,20] Early reports have shown good results in terms of both function and pain relief without the rates of glenoid loosening seen in the previous designs.[21-52]

Indications for Treatment

Our choice of treatment is dictated by numerous factors. The clinical history, physical examination, radiographic findings, and patient expectations must all be taken into account prior to making treatment recommendations and decisions.

In the case of an acute traumatic tear, treatment decisions must be made and implemented rapidly to prevent chronic degenerative changes that may prevent later surgical repair. Partial or small full-thickness tears can be converted to massive tears by acute trauma, such as a fall. These patients may report a long history of minimal to moderate shoulder pain, but may not note significant

disability until the traumatic event. In such a situation, an anteroposterior (AP) radiograph of the shoulder in neutral rotation is used to determine the acromiohumeral distance. An acromiohumeral distance of ≤6 mm is indicative of a long-standing, massive RC tear with fatty infiltration of the infraspinatus. Primary repair of the RC in this case is unlikely to be successful. If the acromiohumeral distance is ≥7 mm, immediate repair of the RC is indicated.

The patient's willingness and ability to tolerate postoperative immobilization and rehabilitation should also be considered. Elderly patients may have difficulty complying with the normal postoperative treatment regimen after cuff repair. Because these patients are frequently not in pain after the pain subsides from the initial injury, nonoperative treatment may be considered. Physiotherapy to maintain ROM and antiinflammatories are helpful. In the event of persistent pain, isolated biceps tenotomy is performed. If disability is an issue and the patient agrees to participate in rehabilitation, cuff repair is considered.

Alternately, a computed tomography (CT) scan or magnetic resonance imaging (MRI) can be used to determine the degree of fatty infiltration of the RC musculature and the reparability of the RC. Goutallier et al[22] graded the fatty infiltration of the muscle using five groups. Stage 0 indicates normal muscle with no fatty changes. In stage 1, there are occasional fatty streaks present. Stage 2 denotes significant fatty infiltration, but there is more muscle than fat present. In stage 3, there is an equal amount of fat and muscle present, and in stage 4, there is more fat than muscle tissue remaining. Stage 3 and 4 changes have been associated with chronic RC tears and a significantly decreased rate of success of cuff repair.[22]

In the case of the chronic RC-deficient shoulder, the functional demands of the patient must be assessed. The patient who uses the arm primarily with the elbow at the side and can compensate for the lack of active elevation by using the contralateral arm is considered to be low demand. Normally, this is the older patient with significant muscular wasting about the shoulder and decreased acromiohumeral distance. If the pain is tolerable, skillful neglect with intermittent physical therapy and medication is frequently the most prudent course of treatment.

Biceps tenotomy may be considered for select patients who have persistent pain and no glenohumeral changes. This works well for posterosuperior tears, but massive tears that also involve the subscapularis have poor results with this technique. This is most likely due to secondary anterior instability of the humeral head with impingement between the coracoid and the lesser tuberosity that can be painful. This procedure normally relieves pain at rest, night pain, and pain that occurs with activities of daily living. Pain that occurs with heavy activity or exercise is not improved. As would be expected, strength and ROM do not show any clinically significant improvement with this technique. Patients who have been able to compensate for the RC tear and regain full motion will maintain this motion after biceps release and do very well. Those who have poor active motion prior to biceps release will show little clinically significant improvement.

The older patient, who complains only of loss of motion, or the pseudoparalytic shoulder, presents different challenges. Palliative procedures, such as biceps tenotomy or cuff débridement are not likely to be successful, as these procedures do nothing to restore a functional cuff mechanism. When the RC tear is long-standing, as evidenced by decreased acromiohumeral distance and fatty infiltration, treatment options available are skillful neglect, muscle transfer, or reverse shoulder arthroplasty. We tend to reserve muscle transfer for those patients who are younger than 70 years old. Elderly patients are treated nonoperatively if they are able to cope with the functional limitations present. If use of the hand at or above the level of the head is required, we have used reverse shoulder arthroplasty with good results.

When the RC tear affects the posterior cuff (infraspinatus and teres minor), patients will present with a loss of ER. The physical examination will typically reveal a positive ER lag sign or dropping sign if the infraspinatus is affected. A positive hornblower's sign will be present in the face of an infraspinatus and teres minor tear. Radiographic signs can be similar to other cuff tears, with long-standing pathology leading to superior migration of the humeral head and a decreased acromiohumeral distance. Once fatty infiltration of the cuff has progressed beyond stage 2, repair is no longer a reasonable option and muscle transfers are considered. If the tear involves both the infraspinatus and the teres minor, latissimus dorsi transfer is required. Again, elderly patients who have low functional demands are treated nonoperatively. Reverse shoulder arthroplasty is not performed in this group, as the prosthesis does nothing to restore ER.

When glenohumeral arthritis is associated with RC deficiency, treatment options are more limited. Glenohumeral changes are always present in the setting of true CTA and may also be seen in association with massive cuff tears and primary osteoarthritis. Nonoperative treatment is always considered as initial treatment. Patients will frequently have significant rest and night pain in addition to loss of function of the shoulder. Activity will only exacerbate these symptoms. Biceps tenotomy and muscle transfers will result in limited pain relief with little functional improvement and are not recommended in these cases. We have employed hemiarthroplasty in the past with acceptable pain relief, but only modest improvements in active motion. Our early experience with reverse shoulder arthroplasty has been extremely encouraging, and we now consider this the treatment of choice for the cuff-deficient shoulder with associated glenohumeral degenerative changes.

Given the short-term follow-up available and the advanced age of most patients reported in the literature, attempts are made to restrict the use of this prosthesis to an older patient population. Patients younger than 60 years of age are encouraged to continue nonoperative therapy, including physical therapy, antiinflammatories, and corticosteroid injections, for as long as possible before reverse arthroplasty.

Fortunately, chronic RC deficiency, with or without glenohumeral changes, is exceedingly rare in young, high-demand patients. If a patient requires use of the arm with the elbow away from the body or for manual labor, glenohumeral arthrodesis is a viable treatment. This is one of the rare indications for which we still routinely employ arthrodesis.

There are several special situations in which the reverse prosthesis is indicated in the younger patient. Revisions of previous hemiarthroplasty or total shoulder arthroplasty frequently result in a poorly functional RC mechanism as it may be damaged during the revision. In addition, severe loss of glenoid and humeral bone stock frequently complicates these already difficult cases. In these situations, the reverse prosthesis is indicated to address the bony and soft tissue deficiencies. Tumor reconstructions also result in significant tissue loss. As in revision surgery, a stable arthrodesis is difficult to obtain after resection of humeral and glenoid bone. This leaves reverse arthroplasty as the only option that may restore some degree of functionality to the shoulder.

Treatment

Cuff Débridement and Biceps Tendon Release

Patient Positioning

The patient is placed in the beach-chair position. We typically employ an operative table that has removable superolateral sections for easy access to the posterior aspect of the shoulder. In lieu of this, a small bump can be placed behind the affected scapula, and the patient can be positioned at the lateral edge of the bed. The arm is draped free, allowing easy positioning during the case.

Surgical Technique

A posterior portal is made approximately 1 cm inferior and 1 cm medial to the posterolateral corner of the acromion. This portal position should allow easy arthroscope placement into the subacromial space and access to the lateral cuff insertion.

Once the presence of a massive and irreparable cuff tear is confirmed, a standard anterolateral working portal is made. The biceps tendon is then sectioned using arthroscopic scissors at the insertion at the supraglenoid tubercle and superior labrum. The tendon is allowed to retract spontaneously out of the glenohumeral joint. In cases where the tendon does not retract, the remaining intraarticular stump is resected.

Synovectomy and bursectomy are performed only to the extent required to provide proper visualization. Acromioplasty is not typically performed.

Postoperative Care

The arm is placed in a simple sling. Passive ROM is allowed beginning on postoperative day one. Active motion is allowed as soon as patient comfort permits. After suture removal, hydrotherapy and a swimming program are begun. Strengthening exercises are avoided as they may result in pain and stiffness.

Reverse Total Shoulder Arthroplasty

Patient Positioning

The patient is placed in the beach-chair position, with the affected shoulder just lateral to the edge of the table. This position should allow hyperextension of the humerus and dislocation of the humeral head. This will permit excellent exposure for the humeral cut and canal preparation. The shoulder is draped so that there is access to the lateral half of the clavicle anteriorly and the lateral half of the scapula posteriorly.

Approach

We routinely use a deltopectoral approach for this procedure, but a superolateral approach can be used as well. We feel that there are several significant advantages to the deltopectoral approach. With this approach, there is no disruption of the deltoid fibers. Although those authors who routinely use the superior approach have not reported significant problems with deltoid function or dehiscence postoperatively, it may be an unnecessary risk when adequate exposure could be obtained through alternative means. Up to 20% of these patients have significant preoperative acromial pathology.[23] In these patients, it would seem counterintuitive to jeopardize the deltoid mechanism further.

The deltopectoral approach is also the standard "workhorse" approach for most shoulder procedures. It is used routinely for anatomical shoulder arthroplasty and is very familiar to most surgeons. This approach affords excellent exposure of the glenoid when combined with an inferior capsular release from the humeral and, in particular, the glenoid sides. These releases are not necessary with a superior approach, but they, along with a partial release of the pectoralis major, are thought to help increase postoperative ROM in those cases of severe arthritis and stiffness.

The deltopectoral approach is an extensile approach, which allows easy access to the anterior humerus. This is especially useful in revision arthroplasty, where humeral osteotomy may be necessary for component extraction. Moreover, identification of the axillary nerve is desirable in these complex cases, and this is best performed through the deltopectoral approach.

Optimal glenoid component placement may be easier through a deltopectoral approach. Difficulties with scapular notching have led many authors to recommend slightly inferior placement of the glenoid component with an inferior tilt, and this is extremely difficult through a superior approach, with the soft tissues and humeral head pushing upward on the glenoid reamers.

The one significant advantage that might be attributed to the superior approach is a lower rate of dislocation.[24] This seems intuitive because the remaining subscapularis muscle is left intact anteriorly.

The deltopectoral incision is begun at the coracoid process and extended distally and laterally for 10 to 15 cm, toward the midpoint of the humerus. The interval is easiest to identify at the most superior and medial portion of the incision. The cephalic vein is left laterally, with the deltoid muscle. Once the interval is opened adequately, the arm is placed in abduction and ER and a Homan retractor is placed over the coracoid process. The arm is returned to full adduction and slight ER, and the pectoralis major insertion is identified and then released along the superior 1 to 2 cm. This exposes the underlying circumflex humeral vessels at the inferior border of the subscapularis, which are ligated using two absorbable sutures.

The coracoacromial ligament is identified and divided just lateral to the coracoid insertion. Release of the fascia from the lateral portion of the conjoined tendon and coracobrachialis muscle allows a small blunt retractor to be placed underneath to expose the underlying subscapularis muscle. The axillary nerve is identified by placing the arm in adduction, slight forward flexion and neutral rotation, and then by following the anterior surface of the subscapularis medially, underneath the conjoined tendon. The nerve is sometimes difficult to see in larger patients, or those with significant fatty tissue surrounding it. In these cases, a larger blunt hand-held retractor (such as a Richardson retractor) is temporarily placed underneath the conjoined tendon to permit location of the nerve. It is then exchanged for a smaller retractor to avoid potential neurovascular complications from prolonged aggressive retraction.

The arm is then placed in abduction and internal rotation (IR) to locate the biceps tendon, which delineates the lateral border of the subscapularis and should lay just medial and deep to the pectoralis major insertion. Dissection using a pair of scissors oriented perpendicular to the tendon usually allows easy entrance into the biceps sheath to identify the tendon if it is still intact. Keeping the arm in the same position, the superior border of the subscapularis is found just behind the tip of the coracoid process.

Once all four borders of the subscapularis have been identified, two stay sutures are placed and the tendon is divided ~1.5 cm medial to insertion on the lesser tuberosity, following the anatomical neck of the humerus.

A humeral head retractor is introduced into the joint to sublux the head posteriorly, and the subscapularis is then released by performing a juxtaglenoid capsulotomy. This is begun by identifying the superior, or semitubular, portion of the subscapularis tendon. Dissecting scissors are slid along the superior tendon edge, releasing any subcoracoid adhesions. The deep surface of the muscle is then bluntly dissected free from the underlying capsule and middle glenohumeral ligament. The capsule and middle glenohumeral ligament are then sectioned, working back inferiorly and medially to the glenoid rim. Next, the previously transected muscle fibers of the inferior subscapularis are found. Lying just posterior to these fibers, which are seen in cross-section, is the inferior glenohumeral ligament. The inferior glenohumeral ligament and capsule are dissected free and sectioned superiorly and medially back to the level of the glenoid. The excursion of the muscle is then tested, and if found to be adequate, the muscle is buried in the subscapularis fossa and protected with a small sponge. If tendon excursion is still inadequate, a blunt instrument can be used to palpate for remaining adhesions on the undersurface of the subscapularis. The muscle is then buried in the subscapularis fossa, and a Kölbel retractor is placed in the fossa to retract the medial structures including the subscapularis muscle, axillary nerve, and conjoined tendon.

At this point, attention is turned to the anterior glenoid, where any remaining labral tissue and subcoracoid bursa is removed. Electrocautery is then used to release the inferior glenoid capsular attachments, past the 6-o'clock position, around to the 7-o'clock position in the right shoulder or the 5-o'clock position in the left shoulder. The release is done directly at the level of the bony attachment and extends medial to the glenoid rim for 2 to 3 mm. This may result in a small release of the triceps insertion, but this is of no functional consequence. So long as the dissection is performed at the bony insertion, there is no danger to the axillary nerve, and in our experience, we have never injured it using this technique. This step is absolutely critical in allowing for proper posterior retraction of the humeral head, and thereby for proper exposure and preparation of the glenoid.

Humeral Preparation

The humeral head retractor is removed and the humeral head is dislocated anteriorly. A sharp Homan retractor can be used to retract any remaining cuff tendon. If the biceps tendon is still intact, it is cut at the level of the glenoid insertion. The intramedullary humeral head cutting guide is then inserted using a starting point determined from the preoperative radiographs. As there is frequently osteonecrosis and deformity of the head, this point can differ from patient to patient, so it is best to simply choose the starting point that gives the most direct in-line access to the medullary canal.

There are two aspects of the cut that can be determined by guide placement; the height and the retroversion. We prefer a minimal head cut to preserve as much humeral length as possible, allowing the prosthesis to be placed in maximal tension. The appropriate retroversion of the cut is

still a matter of considerable debate, and our current strategy is to place the component such that the metaphyseal portion of the prosthesis is contained within the bone of the proximal humerus to the maximum extent possible. This is done without specific regard for the retroversion of the component. In this way, we tend to use the cutting jig as a retroversion gauge rather than a retroversion guide. Frequently, this technique yields retroversion of between 0 and 20 degrees.

Epiphyseal reaming is done using a hemispherical power reamer. The back edge of the reamer is held parallel to the plane of the humeral cut and advanced so that this relationship is maintained. Under normal conditions without significant proximal humeral bone loss, the epiphysis is reamed until the flat edge of the reamer is flush with the surrounding bone.

Diaphyseal reaming is typically done with hand reamers, and trial components are used to ensure proper humeral preparation and fit. The trial components are then removed to allow proper glenoid exposure and preparation.

Glenoid Preparation

Glenoid preparation begins by reinserting a humeral head retractor into the joint, and retracting the head posteriorly. The retractor will usually create a fracture of the thin anterior portion of the humeral metaphysis, what we have termed a *controlled fracture* (**Fig. 10–1**). The fracture has no effect on prosthetic implantation or fixation. This step is only possible if the humeral trial has been removed, because the trial will block efforts to retract the head adequately. An additional Homan retractor is placed superiorly, over the top edge of the glenoid.

The starting point for the peg-hole drill should be several millimeters inferior to the center of the glenoid. Typically, the component is placed as far inferiorly as possible without jeopardizing implant fixation, with an inferior tilt of ~10 degrees.

Glenoid reaming is then performed using the appropriately-sized reamers. Adequate posterior retraction of the humeral head is critical at this point because the reamer is the largest instrument used in glenoid preparation. A selection of several different types of humeral head retractors is helpful if exposure proves difficult.

In osteoporotic bone, there is a tendency for the humeral head to push the reamer anteriorly, causing the central peg of the reamer to cut out of the pilot hole anteriorly. This same effect can also result in excessive anteversion of the glenoid component. In addition, the quality of glenoid bone in these older patients is frequently poor, and care must be taken to not fracture the glenoid while reaming. If the reamer is compressed tightly against the bone first and then started, a large amount of torque is created. If the reamer is started and then gradually pressed against the glenoid face, this torque is lessened, reducing the risk of glenoid fracture.

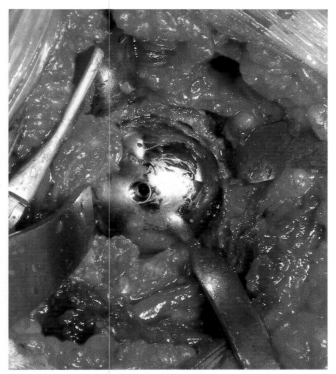

Figure 10–1 Photo showing the controlled fracture of the anterior humeral metaphysis with humeral retractor in place.

Glenoid Implantation

The glenoid baseplate is impacted using an insertion device and fixed in place with screws. Several implants feature fixed or multidirectional locking screws. When possible, two normal compression screws are first placed anteriorly and posteriorly, firmly securing the plate to the underlying glenoid bone. These are followed by locking screws placed superiorly and inferiorly. All screws are placed bicortically when possible.

Care must be taken to be sure that no soft tissue interferes with seating of the glenosphere. Additional posterior or inferior retractors are added when necessary. Most systems include a Morse-taper locking mechanism, which is supplemented with a countersunk safety screw.

Humeral Implantation

Once the glenosphere is in place, the humeral head retractor is removed and the head is dislocated. If there was any remaining subscapularis, three transosseous nonabsorbable sutures are passed to reattach the subscapularis later. The humeral prosthesis is then placed using the retroversion guide to replicate the version of the original humeral cut.

Although trial components are available to test implant stability, they are typically not used. Because the prosthesis

must be placed under significant tension, it is frequently difficult to dislocate once reduced. This can make the removal of trial liners extremely challenging. Instead, the desired thickness of the polyethylene insert is impacted into the metaphyseal component. The reduction is then performed by pulling in-line traction on the arm and pushing posteriorly on the humerus. If this is not possible due to excessive deltoid tension, changing the position of the arm is sometimes helpful. As the humeral component lies anterior to the glenoid, placing of the arm in IR will decrease the profile of the humeral cup that the glenoid must clear to reduce properly. In addition, we have noted that slight forward flexion while pulling traction will sometimes decrease deltoid tension and allow reduction. However, care must be taken to avoid trying to lever the humerus in place, which could result in a periprosthetic fracture. If the reduction is still impossible, a wide, flat instrument, such as an osteotome, can be used as a skid to reduce the prosthesis. The instrument is placed between the glenoid and the humeral cup. The humeral component is then slid posteriorly, along the flat side of the instrument. Once the cup has cleared the glenoid, the instrument is removed allowing the prosthesis to reduce.

After the implant is reduced, the shoulder is taken through a ROM to ensure that there is no significant impingement, and then stability is checked by pulling longitudinal traction. If there is any noticeable pistoning, the polyethylene liner is changed to a thicker size. If the thickest linear is already in place, a modular spacer is placed and the shoulder is reduced and retested. When using the deltopectoral approach, significant pistoning is not acceptable.

Providing that it does not unduly limit ER, the subscapularis is closed using the transosseous sutures. The wound is closed over a drain with absorbable deep and skin sutures.

Postoperative Rehabilitation

Postoperative immobilization consists of a simple sling in IR for one month. Passive ROM and pendulum exercises are begun immediately. After one month, the sling is discarded, and the patient is allowed activity as tolerated. Hydrotherapy is started as soon as possible (usually 2 weeks postoperatively).

Treatment Results

Biceps Tenotomy

Spontaneous rupture of the long head of the biceps tendon occurs frequently as part of the natural history of RC tears.[25] This event is frequently associated with a decrease in pain. Spontaneous ruptures are typically treated nonoperatively with good results.[25–61] Walch et al[26] first proposed isolated biceps tenotomy for pain relief in massive cuff tears. Subsequently, several investigators have also reported on this technique.[27–65] Scheilbel has reported good results in patients with minimal arthritic changes when the tenotomy is combined with an arthroscopic tuberoplasty.[28] Biceps tenotomy has been used for the treatment of biceps tendonitis and instability in the absence of cuff pathology with good results.[29]

Biceps tenotomy has been criticized because of several reports indicating that the tendon of the long head functions as a humeral head depressor.[30–71] It has also been suggested that biceps tenotomy can result in increased subacromial impingement.[25,31] Rupture of the long head of the biceps has also been associated with a 20% loss of forearm supination strength and up to a 20% loss of elbow flexion strength.[32,33] Cosmetic deformity of the biceps muscle is of concern; although some authors have documented its presence, it does not seem to have a great effect on patient satisfaction.[3,34] Distal cramping is frequently seen in spontaneous ruptures or in younger, active, muscular patients; however, this is infrequently noted in tenotomy patients older than 60 years.[27]

Our experience with this technique began in 1988, when the senior author began routinely using this procedure for patients with an irreparable RC with associated upward migration of the humeral head and severe night pain or who were unwilling to undergo the rehabilitation associated with cuff repair. In 2005, the results of 307 patients treated with biceps tenotomy were published with a mean follow-up of almost 5 years.[3] The average preoperative Constant score improved 19.2 points from 48.4 to 67.6. Mean active anterior elevation showed a small, but significant improvement from 153.4 to 164.6 degrees, as most patients had already regained nearly normal motion preoperatively. Eighty-six percent of patients rated their subjective results as good or excellent. Radiographic follow-up did reveal that the mean acromiohumeral distance decreased from 6.6 mm preoperatively to 5.3 mm postoperatively. Furthermore, 24.8% of patients progressed at least one grade on the Hamada classification. Increasing duration of follow-up resulted in progressive narrowing of the acromiohumeral interval and progression of Hamada grade.[3]

Acromioplasty was performed in 110 of these cases. Patients with an acromiohumeral distance of 6 mm or less showed slight decreases in both Constant score and active anterior elevation. When the acromiohumeral distance was greater than 6 mm, results were more favorable. The acromioplasty had no effect on progression of arthritis.

Reverse Total Shoulder Arthroplasty

Functional Results

Because the reverse prosthesis has only been commercially available since 1991, and saw limited usage until recently, the data reported in the current scientific literature is mostly short-term follow-up on relatively small numbers of patients. However, these early reports seem to be very promising. In one of the larger series to date, Sirveaux and colleagues[35] reported on 80 patients with CTA, in a multicenter series at minimum 2-year follow-up. Postoperative Constant scores showed an average increase of 43 points, and active elevation improved 65 to 138 degrees at an average of 44 months postoperatively. Although they noted a 15% complication rate with a 5% rate of revision, 96% complained of little or no residual pain. An intact teres minor was shown to be associated with a better result. DeWilde et al[36] had encouraging results in a small series of 5 patients undergoing revision of an anatomical prosthesis, and again in those patients requiring reconstruction related to tumor resection.[36–45] Rittmeister and Kerschbaumer[37] reported a high complication rate in patients with rheumatoid arthritis, particularly related to a superior approach using an acromial osteotomy. Delloye et al[38] reported on five cases with poor results, having significant problems with loosening, scapular notching, and poor overall outcome. Consequently, this investigator recommended a design change to the prosthesis to address these concerns. In a longer termed investigation, Valenti et al[39] has reported good results in patients with CTA at more than 5-years follow-up with no evidence of progressive glenoid loosening or deterioration of results over time.

Our experience consists of 240 patients who have been treated with Grammont reverse shoulder arthroplasty for a variety of indications, including CTA, massive cuff tear without glenohumeral arthritis, primary osteoarthritis, posttraumatic arthritis, acute proximal humeral fracture, tumor resection, rheumatoid arthritis, and revision of anatomical total shoulder arthroplasty or hemiarthroplasty.[40]

Considering all patients, the average Constant score improved from 22.7 to 59.8. All aspect of the Constant score improved. The average score for pain improved from 3.5 to 12.3. The average score for activity improved from 5.6 to 15.3. The average score for mobility improved from 12.2 to 24.9. The average score for strength improved from 1.5 to 7.0. ROM showed improvement with respect to active elevation and IR; however, no statistically significant improvement was seen for ER. Active elevation improved from a mean of 86 to 137 degrees. Active ER with the arm at the side decreased slightly from a mean of 8 to 6 degrees. Mean IR improved by only one level, from L5 to L4. Ninety-three percent (173) of the 186 patients reported being very satisfied or satisfied with the overall results of their surgeries.

Results did not deteriorate with time. Of the 36 patients with minimum 5-year follow-up included in this patient group, the mean constant score was 59.5, and the mean active elevation was 133.9 degrees. Mean active ER was 6.5 degrees. Mean IR was L3. All 36 patients reported that they were very satisfied or satisfied with their overall results.

When the patients were divided according to reason for reverse shoulder arthroplasty, the best overall results were

Table 10–1   Complications and Frequency among Primary and Revision Reverse Total Shoulder Arthroplasty Patients

Complication	Primary number	%	Revision number	%
Dislocation	8	5.2	7	14.3
Infection	5	3.2	3	6.1
Postoperative humeral fracture	2	1.3	2	6.1
Transient neuropraxia	0	0.0	3	6.1
Scapular spine fracture	1	0.6	1	2.0
Glenoid loosening	2	1.3	0	0.0
Humeral loosening	1	0.6	1	2.0
Glenoid fracture	1	0.6	0	0.0
Humeral spacer unscrewing	0	0.0	1	2.0
Total	20	12.8	18	38.6

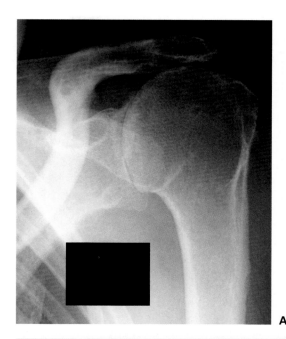

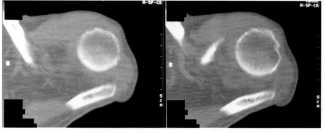

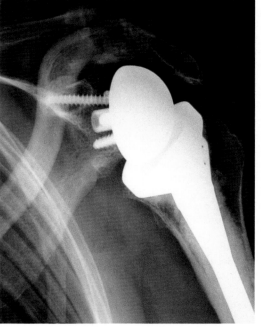

Figure 10–9 (A) Preoperative anteroposterior radiograph and **(B)** computed tomography scan do not demonstrate evidence of scapular spine pathology. **(C)** Two-year follow-up clearly shows scapular spine fracture with significant angulation of the entire acromion.

(12.9 versus 36.7%). The rate of dislocation was nearly triple that of primary surgery (5.2 versus 14.3%). Humeral fracture during humeral implant removal occurred in approximately one fourth of all revisions. Risk of infection was also elevated in the revision population (**Table 10–1**).

Dislocation is of particular concern when discussing reverse shoulder arthroplasty. Several authors have previously reported dislocations, with rates varying from 0 to 31%. DeWilde et al[36] noted exceptionally high dislocation rates in patients undergoing reconstruction after tumor resection and for revision cases.[37–45] Rates for those patients with less complicated pathologies, such as CTA, have been significantly lower. Sirveaux et al[35] noted no instability in 80 patients with CTA after 2 years. Valenti and colleagues had no instance of dislocation in 39 patients with CTA followed for 5 years.[39] Boulahia et al[45] reported only one dislocation in 16 patients with a broad spectrum of underlying diagnoses.

The initial treatment of dislocation is by closed reduction followed by a period of abduction bracing. In recurrent cases or when the prosthesis cannot be closed reduced, open reduction and possible implant revision is indicated. The addition of length to the humeral prosthesis either by increasing the thickness of the polyethylene humeral cup or by using a metallic spacer increases the tension across the joint, and thereby joint stability. In addition, some systems also include a more constrained cup design for these cases (**Fig. 10–9**).

Conclusions

The RC-deficient shoulder is a complex entity that is difficult to treat. This is evidenced by the myriad of treatment options that are available to the surgeon, ranging from nonoperative modalities to arthroplasty and arthrodesis.

There is currently little consensus among shoulder surgeons regarding the uses and indications for these procedures. The relative rarity of this condition means that there are few large studies in the literature, and that most surgeons have little experience with these complications.

In our experience, treatments such as muscle transfers and arthrodesis may be useful in a small subset of carefully selected patients. However, their use is typically limited to very young patients or younger patients with limited active motion.

Biceps tenotomy is a good option for those older patients who have persistent pain, but have preserved active motion, or for older patients who just desire relief of pain. Although concern has been raised over possibly accelerating humeral head migration and progression to CTA, these issues have not been clinically relevant. It is important to remember that tenotomy will not increase motion in a patient who is already stiff; motion must be first regained by judicious use of physical therapy.

The practice of reverse shoulder arthroplasty is still in its infancy and indications are currently expanding. The prosthesis was designed specifically for the cuff-deficient shoulder, and it has had a dramatic impact on our current treatment philosophy. There is sufficient evidence to show that short-term functional results, as measured by the Constant score and clinical exam, are excellent. In addition, patient satisfaction is extremely high; it appears that these gains remain stable, at least for the first 5 years postoperatively.

Early glenoid loosening is no longer a significant problem, with loosening rates approaching those reported for anatomical glenoid components. Short-term complication rates appear to be high, but when the complicated problems to which the prosthesis is being applied are considered, this is not surprising. Preoperative acromial pathology does not require specific treatment, as it seems to have no effect on function, strength or pain relief. Scapular notching, although troublesome on radiographs, has no deleterious effect on functional results and does not progress to glenoid loosening in the short term.

Unfortunately, the list of issues in reverse shoulder arthroplasty yet to be resolved remains very long. This includes items such as the appropriate indications; minimum age of the patients; type of approach, size, and position of the components; appropriate deltoid tension; use of cemented or uncemented components; the importance of subscapularis repair; the use of adjunct muscle transfers, and immobilization and rehabilitation.

References

1. Neer CS II, Craig EV, Fukuda H. Cuff tear arthropathy. J Bone Joint Surg Am 1983;65:1232–1244
2. Hamada K, Fukuda H, Mikasa M, Kobayashi Y. Roentgenographic findings in massive rotator cuff tears a long term observation. Clin Orthop Relat Res 1990;254:92–96
3. Walch G, Edwards TB, Boulahia A, Nové-Josserand L, Neyton L, Szabol I. Arthroscopic tenotomy of the long head of the biceps in the treatment of rotator cuff tears: clinical and radiographic results of 307 cases. J Shoulder Elbow Surg 2005;14:238–246
4. Walch G, Maréchal E, Maupas J, Liotard JP. Traitement chirurgical des ruptures de la coiffe des rotateurs. Facteurs de pronostic. Rev Chir Orthop Reparatrice Appar Mot 1992;78:379–388
5. Fenlin JM, Chase JM, Rushton SA, Frieman BG. Tuberoplasty: creation of an acromiohumeral articulation – a treatment option for massive, irreparable rotator cuff tears. J Shoulder Elbow Surg 2002;11:136–142
6. Rockwood CA, Lyons FR. Shoulder impingement syndrome: diagnosis, radiographic evaluation and treatment with a modified Neer acromioplasty. J Bone Joint Surg Am 1993;75:409–424
7. Rockwood CA, Williams GR, Burkhead WZ. Débridement of degenerative, irreparable lesions of the rotator cuff. J Bone Joint Surg Am 1995;77:857–866
8. Aldridge JM III, Atkinson TS, Mallon WJ. Combined pectoralis major and latissimus dorsi tendon transfer for massive rotator cuff deficiency. J Shoulder Elbow Surg 2004;13:621–629
9. Gerber C, Maquieira G, Espinosa N. Latissimus dorsi transfer for the treatment of irreparable rotator cuff tears. J Bone Joint Surg Am 2006;88:113–120
10. Jost B, Puskas GJ, Lustenberger A, Gerber C. Outcome of pectoralis major transfer for the treatment of irreparable subscapularis tears. J Bone Joint Surg Am 2003;85:1944–1951
11. Arntz CT, Matsen FA III, Jackins S. Surgical management of complex irreparable rotator cuff deficiency. J Arthroplasty 1991;6:363–370
12. Cofield RH, Briggs BT. Glenohumeral arthrodesis: operative and long-term functional results. J Bone Joint Surg Am 1979;61:668–677
13. Diaz JA, Cohen SB, Warren RF, Craig EV, Allen AA. Arthrodesis as a salvage procedure for recurrent anterior instability of the shoulder. J Shoulder Elbow Surg 2003;12:237–241
14. Neer CS II, Watson KC, Stanton FJ. Recent experience in total shoulder replacement. J Bone Joint Surg Am 1982;64:319–337
15. Franklin JL, Barret WP, Jackins SE, Matsen FA. Glenoid loosening in total shoulder arthroplasty. Association with rotator cuff deficiency. J Arthroplasty 1988;3:39–46
16. Sanchez-Sotelo J, Cofield RH, Rowland CM. Shoulder hemiarthroplasty for glenohumeral arthritis associated with severe rotator cuff deficiency. J Bone Joint Surg Am 2001;83:1814–1822
17. Lee DH, Niemann KM. Bipolar shoulder arthroplasty. Clin Orthop Relat Res 1994;304:97–107
18. Coughlin MJ, Morris JM, West WF. The semiconstrained total shoulder arthroplasty. J Bone Joint Surg Am 1979;61:574–581
19. Grammont PM, Baulot E. Delta shoulder prosthesis for rotator cuff rupture. Orthopedics 1993;16:65–68
20. Grammont PM, Trouilloud P, Laffay JP, Deries X. Etude et realisation d'une nouvelle prothèse de l'épaule. Rhumatologie 1987;39:17–22
21. De Buttet M, Bouchon Y, Capon D, Delfosse J. Grammont shoulder arthroplasty for osteoarthritis with massive rotator cuff tears – report of 71 cases [abstract]. J Shoulder Elbow Surg 1997;6:197
22. Goutallier D, Postel JM, Bernageau J, Lavau L, Voisin MC. Fatty muscle degeneration in cuff ruptures. Pre- and postoperative evaluation by CT scan. Clin Orthop Relat Res 1994;304:78–83
23. Mottier F, Wall B, Nové-Josserand L, Galoisy Guibal L, Walch G. L'acromion pathologique dans les prothèses d'épaule inversées. Rev Chirurg Orthop 2007;93:133–161
24. Seebauer L. Reverse prosthesis through a superior approach for cuff tear arthropathy. Tech Shoulder Elbow Surg 2006;7:13–26

25. Neer CS II. Cuff tears, biceps lesions and impingement. In: Neer CS II, ed. Shoulder Reconstruction. Philadelphia, PA: WB Saunders; 1990:73–77

26. Walch G, Boulahia A, Levigne C, Nové-Josserand L. Arthroscopic tenotomy of the biceps tendon as a salvage procedure for non-repairable rotator cuff tear. Paper presented at: 7th International Conference on Surgery of the Shoulder; October 5–8, 1998; Sydney, Australia

27. Kelly AM, Drakos MC, Fealy S, Taylor SA, O'Brien SJ. Arthroscopic release of the long head of the biceps tendon: functional outcome and clinical results. Am J Sports Med 2005;33:208–213

28. Scheibe IM, Lichtenberg S, Habermeyer P. Reversed arthroscopic subacromial decompression for massive rotator cuff tears. J Shoulder Elbow Surg 2004;13:272–278

29. Gill TJ, McIrvin E, Mair SD, Hawkins RJ. Results of biceps tenotomy for treatment of pathology of the long head of the biceps brachii. J Shoulder Elbow Surg 2001;10:247–249

30. Flatow EL, Raimondo RA, Kelkar R, et al. Active and passive restraints against superior humeral translation: the contributions of the rotator cuff, biceps tendon, and the coracoacromial arch. Paper presented at: 12th Annual Open Meeting of the American Shoulder and Elbow Surgeons; February 25, 1996; Atlanta, GA

31. Neer CS II. Treatment of impingement lesions of the biceps. In: Neer CS II, ed. Shoulder Reconstruction. Philadelphia, PA: WB Saunders; 1990:134–137

32. Mariani E, Cofield RH, Askew LJ, Li G, Chao EYS. Rupture of the tendon of the long head of the biceps brachii: surgical versus nonsurgical treatment. Clin Orthop Relat Res 1988;228:233–239

33. Soto-Hall R, Stroor JH. Treatment of ruptures of the long head of biceps brachii. Am J Orthop 1960;2:192–193

34. Osbahr DC, Diamond AB, Speer KP. The cosmetic appearance of the biceps muscle after long-head tenotomy versus tenodesis. Arthroscopy 2002;18:483–487

35. Sirveaux F, Favard L, Oudet D, Huguet D, Walch G, Molé D. Grammont inverted total shoulder arthroplasty in the treatment of glenohumeral osteoarthritis with massive rupture of the cuff. J Bone Joint Surg Br 2004;86-B:388–395

36. De Wilde L, Mombert M, Van Petegem P, Verdonk R. Revision of shoulder replacement with a reversed shoulder prosthesis (Delta III): report of five cases. Acta Orthop Belg 2001;67:348–353

37. Rittmeister M, Kerschbaumer F. Grammont reverse total shoulder arthroplasty in patients with rheumatoid arthritis and nonreconstructible rotator cuff lesions. J Shoulder Elbow Surg 2001;10:17–22

38. Delloye C, Joris D, Colette A, Eudier A, Dubuc JE. Complications mécaniques de la prothèse totale inverse de l'épaule. Rev Chirur Orthop 2002;88:410–414

39. Valenti Ph, Boutens D, Nerot C. Delta 3 reversed prosthesis for arthritis with massive rotator cuff tear: long term results (> 5 years). In: Walch G, Boileau P, Molé D, eds. 2000 Shoulder Prosthesis... Two to Ten Year Follow-Up. Montpellier, France: Sauramps Medical;2001:253–260

40. Wall B, Walch G, Nové-Josserand L, Edwards TB. Results of reverse shoulder arthroplasty according to etiology [abstract]. Paper presented at: American Academy of Orthopedic Surgeons 2006 Annual Meeting; March 22–26, 2006; Chicago, IL

41. Werner C, Steinmann P, Gilbart M, Gerber C. Treatment of painful pseudoparesis due to irreparable rotator cuff dysfunction with the Delta III reverse-ball-and-socket total shoulder prosthesis. J Bone Joint Surg Am 2005;87:1476–1486

42. Dennis D, Ferlic D, Clayton M. Acromial stress fractures associated with cuff-tear arthropathy. J Bone Joint Surg Am 1986;68:937–940

43. Frankle M, Siegal S, Pupello D, Saleem A, Mighell M, Vasey M. The reverse shoulder prosthesis for glenohumeral arthritis associated with severe rotator cuff deficiency. J Bone Joint Surg Am 2005;87:1697–1705

44. De Wilde L, Sys G, Julien Y, Van Ovost E, Poffyn B, Trouilloud P. The reversed Delta shoulder prosthesis in reconstruction of the proximal humerus after tumour resection. Acta Orthop Belg 2003;69:495–500

45. Boulahia A, Edwards TB, Walch G, Baratta R. Early results of a reverse design prosthesis in the treatment of arthritis of the shoulder in elderly patients with a large rotator cuff tear. Orthopedics 2002;25:129–133

46. Gilbart MK, Pirki C, Gerber C. Complications associated with the Delta III reverse ball-and-socket shoulder prosthesis. Paper presented at: International Conference of Shoulder Surgeons; 2004;Washington, DC

47. VanHove B, Beugnies A. Grammont's reverse shoulder prosthesis for rotator cuff arthropathy. A retrospective study of 32 cases. Acta Orthop Belg May 3–5, 2004;70:219–225

48. Jacobs R, DeBeer P, De Smet L. Treatment of rotator cuff arthropathy with a reversed Delta shoulder prosthesis. Acta Orthop Belg 2001;67:344–347

49. Wall B, Jouve F, Nové-Josserand L, Walch G. Complications and revisions in reverse shoulder arthroplasty [abstract]. Paper presented at: American Academy of Orthopedic Surgeons 2006 Annual Meeting; March 22–26, 2006; Chicago, IL

50. Aoki M, Okamura K, Fukushima S, Takahashi T, Ogino T. Transfer of latissimus dorsi for irreparable rotator-cuff tears. J Bone Joint Surg Br 1996;78:761–766

51. Gerber C. Latissimus dorsi transfer for the treatment of irreparable tears of the rotator cuff. Clin Orthop Relat Res 1992;275:152–160

52. Miniaci A, MacLeod M. Transfer of the latissimus dorsi muscle after failed repair of a massive tear of the rotator cuff. A two to five-year review. J Bone Joint Surg Am 1999;81:1120–1127

53. Warner JJ, Parsons IM IV. Latissimus dorsi tendon transfer: a comparative analysis of primary and salvage reconstruction of massive, irreparable rotator cuff tears. J Shoulder Elbow Surg 2001;10:514–521

54. Cofield RH. Total shoulder arthroplasty with the Neer prosthesis. J Bone Joint Surg Am 1984;66:899–906

55. Hawkins RJ, Neer CS II. A functional analysis of shoulder fusions. Clin Orthop Relat Res 1987;223:65–76

56. Richards RR, Sherman RM, Hudson AR, Waddell JP. Shoulder arthrodesis using a pelvic-reconstruction plate: a report of eleven cases. J Bone Joint Surg Am 1988;70:416–421

57. Richards RR, Waddell JP, Hudson AR. Shoulder arthrodesis for the treatment of brachial plexus palsy. Clin Orthop Relat Res 1985;198:250–258

58. Rybka V, Raunio P, Vainio K. Arthrodesis of the shoulder in rheumatoid arthritis: a review of forty-one cases. J Bone Joint Surg Br 1979;61:155–158

59. Wick M, Müller EJ, Ambacher T, Hebler U, Muhr G, Kutscha-Lissberg F. Arthrodesis of the shoulder after septic arthritis: long-term results. J Bone Joint Surg Br 2003;85:666–670

60. Williams GR, Rockwood CA. Hemiarthroplasty in rotator cuff-deficient shoulders. J Shoulder Elbow Surg 1996;5:362–367

61. Zuckerman JD, Scott AJ, Gallagher MA. Hemiarthroplasty for cuff tear arthropathy. J Shoulder Elbow Surg 2000;9:169–172

62. Sarris IK, Papadimitriou NG, Sotereanos DG. Bipolar hemiarthroplasty for chronic rotator cuff tear arthropathy. J Arthroplasty 2003;18:169–173

63. Worland RL, Jessup DE, Arredondo J, Warburton KJ. Bipolar shoulder arthroplasty for rotator cuff arthropathy. J Shoulder Elbow Surg 1997;6:512–515

64. Fenlin JM. Total glenohumeral joint replacement. Orthop Clin North Am 1975;6:565–583

65. Gerard P, LeBlanc JP, Rousseau B. Une prothèse totale d'épaule. Chirurgie 1973;99:655–663

66. Lettin AWF, Copeland SA, Scales JT. The Stanmore total shoulder replacement. J Bone Joint Surg Br 1982;64:47–51

67. Post M, Haskell SS, Jablon M. Total shoulder replacement with a constrained prosthesis. J Bone Joint Surg Am 1980;62:327–335

68. Post M, Jablon M, Miller H, Singh M. Constrained total shoulder joint replacement: a critical review. Clin Orthop Relat Res 1979;144:135–150

69. Post M, Jablon M. Constrained total shoulder joint replacement: long-term follow-up observations. Clin Orthop Relat Res 1983;173:109–116

70. Post M. Constrained arthroplasty of the shoulder. Orthop Clin North Am 1987;18:455–462

71. De Wilde LF, Van Ovost E, Uyttendaele D, Verdonk R. Résultats d'une prothèse d'épaule inversée après résection pour tumeur de l'humérus proximal. Rev Chir Orthop Reparatrice Appar Mot 2002;88:373–378

72. McMaster PE. Tendon and muscle ruptures: clinical and experimental studies on the causes and location of subcutaneous ruptures. J Bone Joint Surg Am 1933;15:705–722

73. Sethi N, Wright R, Yamaguchi K. Disorders of the long head of the biceps tendon. J Shoulder Elbow Surg 1999;8:644–654

74. Waugh RL, Hathcock TA, Elliot JL. Ruptures of muscles and tendons: with particular reference to rupture (or elongation of long tendon) of biceps brachii with report of fifty cases. Surgery 1949;25:370–392

75. Kempf JF, Gleyze P, Bonnomet F, et al. A multicenter study of 210 rotator cuff tears treated by arthroscopic acromioplasty. Arthroscopy 1999;15:56–66

76. Klinger HM, Spahn G, Baums MH, Stecke IH. Arthroscopic debridement of irreparable massive rotator cuff tears: a comparison of debridement alone and combined procedure with biceps tenotomy. Acta Chir Belg 2005;105:297–301

77. Itoi E, Kuechle DK, Newman SR, Morrey BF, An KN. Stabilizing function of the biceps in stable and unstable shoulders. J Bone Joint Surg Br 1993;75:546–550

78. Kumar VP, Satku K, Balasubramaniam P. The role of the long head of biceps brachii in the stabilization of the long head of the humerus. Clin Orthop Relat Res 1989;244:172–175

79. Rodosky MW, Harner CD, Fu FH. The role of the long head of the biceps muscle and superior glenoid labrum in anterior stability of the shoulder. Am J Sports Med 1994;22:121–130

11 Treating the Rotator Cuff–Deficient Shoulder: The Mayo Clinic Experience

John W. Sperling and Robert H. Cofield

There has been an evolution in the treatment of rotator cuff arthropathy (RCA) at the Mayo Clinic (Rochester, MN). There was a brief experience with constrained and semiconstrained designs in the 1970s and 1980s. However, the predominant treatment for the last 25 years has been hemiarthroplasty. Recently, there has been incorporation of a reverse prosthesis design for the treatment of select patients with cuff tear arthropathy (CTA). Our purpose in this chapter is to discuss the Mayo Clinic experience in treating RCA with shoulder arthroplasty. The results, risk factors for an unsatisfactory outcome, and rates of failure will be reviewed.

Hemiarthroplasty (Humeral Head Replacement)

In the late 1970s, there was recognition of a group of patients who had destruction of glenohumeral cartilage in association with severe RC tearing. This was often associated with instability as well as some degree of bone loss. Neer and coworkers[1] have described a CTA to better characterize this syndrome.

In 1986, Brownlee and Cofield reported on 20 shoulder replacements performed for CTA between 1976 and 1982.[2] Sixteen shoulder arthroplasties were available for review at a mean of 4 years following surgery. A humeral head replacement without a glenoid component was performed in four shoulders. In these patients, there was a reduction of pain in all shoulders, but there was little change in active motion. There were no reoperations among these four shoulders. However, in the remaining 12 shoulders that had placement of a glenoid component, revision was needed for glenoid component problems in three shoulders. This group was reviewed in 1991, and no substantive changes had occurred over time.[3]

The results of shoulder hemiarthroplasty for RCA at the Mayo Clinic in a series of 33 shoulders, followed for an average of 5 years, was recently reviewed by Sanchez-Sotelo and colleagues.[4] Eleven shoulders had undergone between one and four previous procedures, including an acromioplasty in eight shoulders. Shoulder hemiarthroplasty was associated with significant pain relief (**Fig. 11–1** and **Fig. 11–2**). However, at the most recent follow-up, 9 patients (27%) had moderate pain at rest or pain with activity. The mean active elevation improved from 72 to 91 degrees ($p = 0.008$), mean internal rotation improved from L3 to L1 ($p = 0.02$), and mean active external rotation improved from 36 to 41 degrees (not significant). According to Neer's limited goals criteria, successful results were achieved in 22 cases (67%). However, most patients were satisfied with the outcome of the surgery and only four shoulders were subjectively considered to be the same or worse than before the operation. Two factors were associated with a less satisfactory outcome: prior subacromial decompression and the extent of proximal migration of the humeral head.

The experience with hemiarthroplasty for RCA revealed that a less satisfactory outcome should be expected in patients with prior violation of the coracoacromial arch. The use of either small humeral head sizes in an attempt to

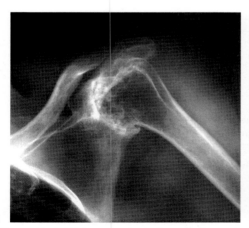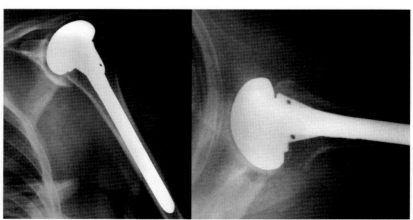

A   B

Figure 11–1 **(A)** Preoperative radiograph demonstrates rotator cuff arthropathy with central glenoid erosion. The patient had active elevation to 100 degrees and severe pain. **(B)** Postoperatively, the patient had mild pain and 110 degrees of elevation.

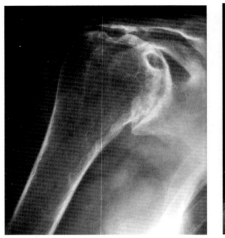 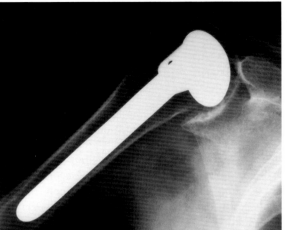

Figure 11–2 (A) Patient with rheumatoid arthritis and massive rotator cuff tear. Preoperatively, she had severe pain and active elevation to 70 degrees. **(B)** One-year postoperative, she had no pain and active elevation to 90 degrees.

facilitate reconstruction of the cuff or large sizes to maximize joint stability did not seem to be justified.

Constrained and Semi-constrained Total Shoulder Arthroplasty

There was a strong initial interest in the design of total shoulder prostheses that included a constrained or a ball-in-socket design. Unfortunately, the frequency of complications was found to be extraordinarily high. In addition, these complications were often quite serious and included dislocations, component material failure, or component loosening, most of which necessitated major revision surgery. As an alternative to a completely captive ball-in-socket arrangement, hooded or semiconstrained glenoid components were designed as a part of a prosthetic system.

Early in our experience with total shoulder arthroplasty, we became involved to a limited extent with the use of constrained total shoulder arthroplasties in patients with various forms of glenohumeral arthritis. One of the early designs of a constrained total shoulder arthroplasty was developed by Dr. William Bickel[5] at the Mayo Clinic. The intent was to incorporate the low-friction concept of Charnley and for the glenoid component to be entirely encased within the glenoid process of the scapula to maximize the area of bone–cement contact.[5] Unfortunately, this experience was similar to the experience of others and to our experience with the Stanmore shoulder prosthesis (**Table 11–1**). Significant complications were very common. Most notably, these included glenoid loosening and instability. Revision surgery was necessary in 12 of the 27 shoulders (44%). Our experience was better with the Michael Reese design, but later failures occurred (largely glenoid loosening). This implant was subsequently removed from the market.

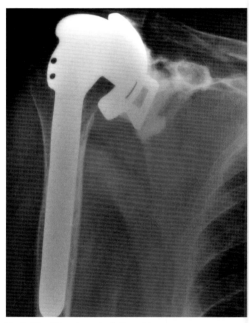

Figure 11–3 The Neer hooded glenoid component.

Table 11–1   Mayo Clinic's Results Using Constrained Total Shoulder Replacement

	Followup		Active	
Prosthesis	**Years**	**Shoulders**	**Abduction**	**Revision**
Bickel	12	12	95	8
Stanmore	9	9	93	4
Michael Reese	7	6	73	0

Fifteen shoulders did not have intervening revision surgery and were available for analysis more than 2 years after their initial surgical procedure. As in other series, satisfactory pain relief usually occurred, but return of active abduction was disappointing, averaging between one-third and one-half normal. Using a rating system similar to Neer's published criteria, there were no excellent results, 5 satisfactory results, and 22 unsatisfactory results.[6]

An additional design that was used at the Mayo Clinic was the Neer hooded glenoid component. This glenoid component was designed with a metal backed keel and was oversized to compensate for superior subluxation associated with RCA. Nwakama and Cofield[7] reviewed the results of seven shoulders that underwent this procedure. Six of the seven shoulders had an unsatisfactory outcome. Two patients required revision surgery for subluxation or glenoid loosening (**Fig. 11–3**).

Treatment Algorithm

The initial treatment for patients with RCA includes activity modification, simple nonsteroidal antiinflammatory medications, a gentle home physiotherapy program including pain relieving measures, gentle stretching, and light strengthening. In addition, corticosteroid injections may be helpful. When patients have failed these nonoperative measures, one can then consider operative intervention.

If there is considerable irregularity of movement, a form of crepitus, and the arthritis is moderate, arthroscopic debridement may be considered. However, this procedure is not commonly needed. For those patients who might be considered surgical candidates, the tendency is to perform a hemiarthroplasty when the humeral head is stable beneath the acromial arch, when the glenoid erosion is substantial, or when there is active elevation to $\geq$60 or 70 degrees. In addition, among younger patients and those who actively use their shoulders and arms, hemiarthroplasty is typically performed.

The reverse prosthesis is used more frequently when there is anterosuperior escape of the proximal humerus; when the glenoid is intact, or relatively so; or when the patient has pseudoparalysis, barely being able to raise the arm away from the side. The reverse prosthesis is most appropriate for elderly patients and those who are sedentary.

Summary

Early experience with constrained or semi-constrained designs for the treatment of RCA resulted in a high complication and failure rate. Humeral head replacement has been found to have a moderate chance of good to excellent pain relief, minimal improvement in motion, and a low rate of mechanical failure. Risk factors for an unsatisfactory outcome with hemiarthroplasty include a prior subacromial decompression and significant superior subluxation. The reverse prosthesis has provided a new option to treat patients with RCA, particularly those patients with anterosuperior escape. The early experience with a reverse prosthesis has been encouraging; however, longer follow-up will be necessary to determine the durability of this prosthesis.

References

1. Neer CS, Craig EV, Fukuda H. Cuff-tear arthropathy. J Bone Joint Surg Am 1983;65:1232–1244
2. Brownlee RC, Cofield RH. Shoulder replacement in cuff tear arthropathy. Orthop Trans 1986;10:230
3. Lohr JF, Cofield RH, Uhthoff HK. Glenoid component loosening in cuff tear arthropathy. J Bone Joint Surg Br 1991;73-B(Suppl):106
4. Sanchez-Sotelo J, Cofield RH, Rowland CM. Shoulder hemiarthroplasty for glenohumeral arthritis associated with severe rotator cuff deficiency. J Bone Joint Surg Am 2001;12:1814–1822
5. Cofield RH, Stauffer RN. The Bickel glenohumeral arthroplasty. In: Morrey, BF (ed) Conference on Joint Replacement in the Upper Limb. Bury St Edmunds, UK: Institute of Mechanical Engineering Publications; 1977:15–25
6. Cofield RH. Results and complications of shoulder arthroplasty. In: BF Morrey, ed. Reconstructive Surgery of the Joints. 2nd ed. New York, NY: Churchill Livingstone; 1996: 773–787
7. Nwakama AC, Cofield RH, Kavanagh BF, Loehr JF. Semiconstrained total shoulder arthroplasty for glenohumeral arthritis and massive rotator cuff tearing. J Shoulder Elbow Surg 2000;9(4):302–307

12 Treating the Rotator Cuff–Deficient Shoulder: The Columbia University Experience

John-Erik Bell, Sara L. Edwards, and Louis U. Bigliani

History

The Legacy of Harrison L. McLaughlin

The New York Orthopaedic Hospital, located within New York Presbyterian Hospital, Columbia Campus, in upper Manhattan, has supported the work of great leaders in shoulder surgery throughout the 20th century, a privilege that continues today. The pedigree of the Shoulder Service is extensive; it has its roots within the renowned Fracture Service, established by Dr. William Darrach. Harrison Lloyd McLaughlin, M.D., F.A.C.S. (**Fig. 12–1**) began his medical career on the Fracture Service in 1935 under Darrach and established himself as a pioneer in the study of the rotator cuff (RC) and its pathology.[1] With seminal studies on lesions of the RC and their surgical repair published in the

1940s and 1950s, McLaughlin staked his position as an innovative thinker in the pathology and treatment of RC disease.[2–5] Although best known for his contributions to the field of shoulder instability, and, in particular, posterior dislocation, with an operative procedure bearing his name, his theories on RC pathology have served as the foundation for successive leaders of the Columbia Shoulder Service.[2] In his report on 100 consecutive patients and their long-term follow-up, McLaughlin wrote, "Operative experiences soon demonstrated that no two tendon ruptures were similar or amenable to identical repair techniques, that each required a plastic tenorrhaphy suited to its own original characteristics . . ." He realized that the three prerequisites to a successful repair included "1) The snug apposition of healthy to healthy tissue without tension at the site of repair. 2) The restoration of continuity between the short rotator muscle bellies and the humerus. 3) The restoration of a smooth surface for articulation with the acromion. . ." He also suggested the impingement phenomenon in which the RC and bursa are compressed between the humeral head and acromion, which has been expanded upon by following leaders of the Columbia Shoulder Service, Drs. Charles S. Neer and Louis U. Bigliani.[2]

The Legacy of Charles S. Neer, II

Charles S. Neer, M.D. (**Fig. 12–2**) is considered by many to be the father of modern shoulder surgery. Dr. Neer developed the first widely used prosthetic shoulder replacement, established the most commonly used classification of proximal humerus fractures, and advanced the management of shoulder instability.[3–8] Neer created the first shoulder fellowship in the world and initiated the great legacy of the Columbia Shoulder Service. Many leaders in shoulder surgery around the world have either trained under Neer and with those whom he trained. With respect to the RC-deficient shoulder, Neer first described the radiographic and clinical features of arthritis associated with massive RC tear in 1977 and, in 1983, Neer coined the term *cuff tear arthropathy* in his classic paper on the subject.[4,5]

Neer reported on 26 patients with cuff tear arthropathy (CTA) who underwent surgical reconstruction with total shoulder replacement at Columbia between 1975 and 1983.[4] He described their symptoms as "remarkably similar," consisting of "long-standing and progressively increas-

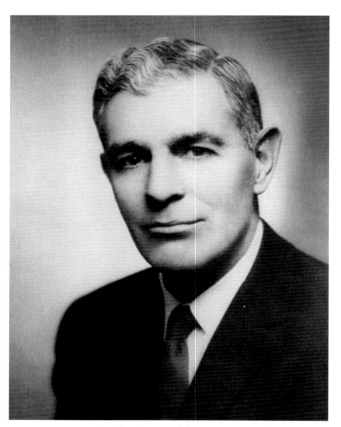

Figure 12–1 Harrison Lloyd McLaughlin, M.D., F.A.C.S.

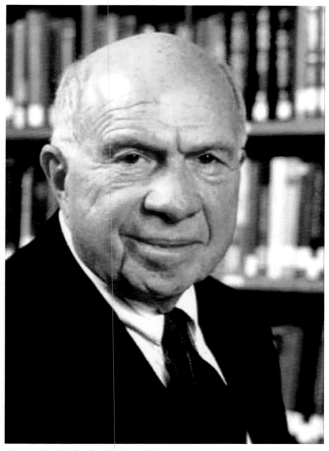

Figure 12–2 Charles S. Neer, M.D.

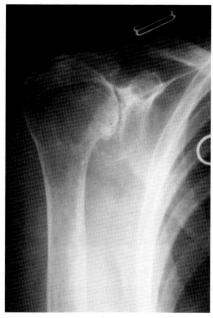

Figure 12–3 Anteroposterior radiograph of one of Dr. Neer's cuff tear arthropathy patients. Note superior head migration and corresponding loss of the acromiohumeral interval, superior glenoid erosion creating a biconcave glenoid, erosion of the acromion, and rounding off of the greater tuberosity.

ing pain that was worse at night, was exacerbated by use and activity, and was made more intense by movement of the humerus against the scapula . . . and the patients complained of inability to elevate or externally rotate the shoulder." Physical examination revealed swelling of the shoulder resulting from synovial fluid communicating between the glenohumeral joint and the subacromial space (the "fluid sign"), atrophy of the supraspinatus and infraspinatus muscles with corresponding weakness of external rotation (ER) and abduction, decreased active elevation (only 2 patients of 26 could actively elevate above 90 degrees), and crepitus at the glenohumeral joint line. Radiographic findings were described as "characteristic," consisting of collapse of the proximal humerus, instability of the glenohumeral joint, loss of the acromiohumeral distance, and erosion of the superior glenoid, inferior acromion, coracoid, distal clavicle, and greater tuberosity (**Fig. 12–3**).

At the time of surgery, Neer found a large, complete RC tear in all patients, involving the supraspinatus in all, the infraspinatus in all but one, and often involving the subscapularis and teres minor muscles as well. Instability was also common, with 14 shoulders exhibiting passive dislocation and 12 shoulders demonstrating fixed dislocation. Dramatic cartilage loss was noted, and radiographic find-

ings of coracoacromial arch erosions were confirmed at surgery. Neer also performed histologic studies, and found that the humeral head became covered with a disordered fibrous membrane, with the underlying bone osteoporotic and hypervascular. He also found areas at points of fixed contact with the scapula that resembled changes seen in osteoarthritis with complete loss of articular cartilage and subchondral sclerosis. Finally, he found fragments of articular cartilage in subsynovial layers which resembled those found in neuropathic joints and hypothesized that these were the products of instability and subsequent abnormal trauma to the articular surfaces.

Neer's theory regarding the etiology of CTA was also put forth in this seminal paper.[4] He proposed the hypothesis that the reason this condition only affects the glenohumeral joint and not other joints is because of the shoulder's unique dependence on the soft tissue for stability and relative lack of bony constraint. He hypothesized that both nutritional and mechanical factors are important in the development of CTA:

Nutritional factors imposed by the massive tear include loss of a closed joint space and impaired movement of the glenohumeral joint. The loss of a closed joint space with leaking synovial fluid under reduced pressure would be expected to deter the perfusion of nutrients into the articular cartilage. Joint inactivity has been shown to lead to structural alterations in articular cartilage as well as to biochemical changes in the water and glycosaminoglycan content of the cartilage and capsule. Both then, loss of a closed joint space and inactivity, are thought to contribute to the atrophy of the articular cartilage of the humeral head. Inactivity is also thought to cause disuse osteoporosis of the subchondral bone, in accordance with Wolff's law, which may eventually lead to collapse of the subchondral bone . . . The mechanical factors include gross instability of the humeral head on the glenoid as well as upward migration of the head against the acromion and acromioclavicular joint. Loss of the stabilizing functions of the long head of the biceps following rupture or displacement of its tendon as well as of the RC contribute to at least two types of instability. Anterior and posterior subluxations and dislocations produce abnormal trauma and injury to the articular surfaces of the humeral head and glenoid. Eventually the incongruous head may erode through the glenoid into the coracoid process. The upward instability and upward migration of the head escalate the previously described process of subacromial impingement.[6] Impingement wear erodes the anterior part of the acromion, the acromioclavicular joint, and the outer part of the clavicle. Instability of the head seems to be essential for the development of its collapse.[4]

Neer treated his 26 patients with total shoulder arthroplasty (**Fig. 12–4**), which is now considered to be less preferable than hemiarthroplasty due to early glenoid loosening from eccentric loading and increased lateral offset.[7–14] He remarked, "surgical reconstruction of these shoulders is especially difficult." Nevertheless, he found that only one of the 26 patients did not consider the procedure helpful. His paper first describing the entity of CTA laid the groundwork for many subsequent investigations and treatments for this previously unrecognized condition.

One such subsequent investigation performed at Columbia is that of Pollock et al.[7] In this study, 30 shoulders with glenohumeral arthritis and RC deficiency, which had undergone prosthetic replacement, were retrospectively reviewed at an average of 41 months follow-up. Of these, 19 had undergone hemiarthroplasty and 11 had undergone total shoulder arthroplasty. All had an attempt at RC repair. Both total shoulder arthroplasty and hemiarthroplasty had similar levels of pain relief and patient satisfaction. The most interesting finding was that, despite similar levels of pain relief, the group undergoing hemiarthroplasty displayed a significant improvement in active forward elevation (+52 versus +2 degrees) postoperatively compared with those undergoing total shoulder arthroplasty. The surgeons felt that hemiarthroplasty afforded greater ease of RC repair because the lateral offset of the humerus was decreased relative to that of total shoulder arthroplasty, and that this technical factor might be responsible for improved postoperative active elevation. Because of these findings, hemiarthroplasty has been the procedure of choice at Columbia for CTA over the past decade.

Treatment of Cuff Tear Arthropathy

Overview

At Columbia, a significant number of patients with CTA are treated every year. These patients are approached in a systematic way, utilizing multiple treatment modalities. The most important variables that factor into our treatment decision include patient age, functional status, pain level, active and passive range of motion, and findings on preoperative imaging studies. The first decision to make is whether the patient is better suited for nonoperative treatment or is a candidate for surgical reconstruction. Typically, all patients with CTA have a trial of nonoperative treatment, consisting of antiinflammatory medications and physical therapy to strengthen the remaining fibers of the teres minor and subscapularis in an attempt to recreate a force-couple to restore some active elevation to the shoulder. For patients in reasonable health who fail nonoperative treatment, we recommend surgical reconstruction of the shoulder. For patients with multiple comorbidities for whom surgery is perilous, we continue with definitive nonoperative treatment.

Once it has been decided that surgery is indicated, we must decide which prosthesis or procedure is indicated. Potential solutions to this problem include débridement, open RC repair with or without tendon transfers, arthrodesis, resection arthroplasty, and prosthetic arthroplasty. Prosthetic choices include hemiarthroplasty designs such as resurfacing implants, traditional stemmed components,

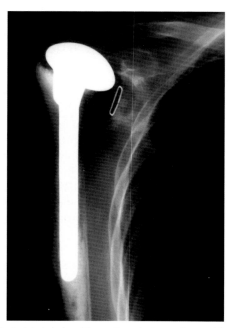

Figure 12–4 A total shoulder arthroplasty performed by Dr. Neer for the patient from Fig. 12–3. Note the superior migration of the humeral head and the subsequent eccentric loading of the superior aspect of the glenoid prosthesis.

and newer expanded heads that cover the greater tuberosity. At Columbia, Neer had extensive experience with traditional total shoulder arthroplasty for CTA as well as enlarged glenoid components that increase superior constraint (**Fig. 12–5**).[5] Traditional glenoid replacement has been subsequently shown to result in unacceptably high rates of failure secondary to superior humeral head migration, glenoid loosening, and poor functional results.[7,8]

In recent years, there has been renewed enthusiasm for the reverse total shoulder prosthesis based on Grammont's design improvements detailed elsewhere in this textbook. At Columbia, several dozen reverse total shoulder arthroplasties have been performed with promising early results. The most important factor in the success of this implant is choosing the correct indications.

Hemiarthroplasty remains an excellent option for patients with CTA if the right indications exist.[7,9–20] While the reverse prosthesis is promising and seems attractive, it may not be indicated in all cases. We approach this procedure with both excitement and caution due to reports of high rates of short-term complications by experienced surgeons in Europe and in the United States.[10,11] At Columbia, this new technology is utilized for very specific and narrow indications with good short-term results. The ideal indication for the reverse prosthesis is for patients over the age of 70 with both pseudoparalysis and advanced CTA. It is also indicated for more complex reconstructive situations, including revision of failed hemiarthroplasty for fracture with tuberosity nonunion, and other revision situations without a functional RC; however, results for such revision cases have been less consistent. We do not utilize this prosthesis in patients who have greater than 90 degrees of active forward elevation, those under age 70 or who anticipate heavy activity levels postoperatively, those with poor glenoid bone stock, or in those who have an incompetent deltoid. Hemiarthroplasty is indicated in those patients with active forward elevation above 90 degrees.

Our contraindications to hemiarthroplasty include deltoid deficiency and a disrupted coracoacromial arch with anterosuperior escape.[12,13]

Hemiarthroplasty

The patient is positioned ~30 degrees upright in a beach-chair position with a short arm board under the affected extremity. The shoulder is exposed through a standard deltopectoral approach. The proximal one third of the pectoralis major tendon is released with cautery. The subscapularis is carefully released as far lateral as possible, so that as much length as possible can be achieved in the subscapularis tendon. The goal of subscapularis reconstruction is to advance it as far superiorly as possible, often to the anterior part of the greater tuberosity. The subscapularis is reattached more medially at the surgical neck cut. This will also add length. It is critical to preserve the coracoacromial ligament to maintain the coracoacromial arch in the RC-deficient shoulder. The biceps tendon is usually ruptured, but if present it should be preserved. The head is then dislocated by positioning the extremity in adduction, extension, and ER. We use the Zimmer Bigliani–Flatow shoulder arthroplasty system (Zimmer, Inc., Warsaw, IN). The canal is reamed until there is a palpable tight fit, then the reamer is used to align the proximal humerus cutting jig. The head is resected at the level of the articular margin in ~30 degrees of retroversion. In CTA, retroversion between 30 to 40 degrees is preferred to minimize anterosuperior subluxation. It is sometimes difficult to determine where the articular margin stops and the greater tuberosity begins because the cartilage is absent and the greater tuberosity has been eroded significantly. In these situations, preoperative templating is critical, using the contralateral shoulder as a guide if possible. The rule of thumb is to resect less rather than more of the humeral head. We frequently use

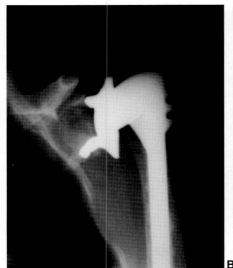 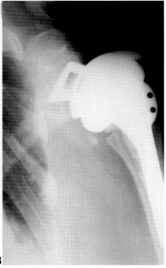

A   B

Figure 12–5 Examples of semiconstrained total shoulder replacements performed by Dr. Neer for cuff-tear arthropathy. **(A)** A 200% glenoid component; **(B)** a 600% glenoid component.

a stem proximally coated with trabecular metal, allowing bone ingrowth. The majority of patients are osteoporotic, or have otherwise poor bone quality, with excessively capacious canal diameters, and require proximal cementing technique for increased axial and rotational stability.

We prefer an attempt at RC repair if possible. Frequently, the cuff will be irreparable, but if some posterior cuff can be repaired, it can function in concert with the subscapularis to obtain a "force-couple" which may allow the patient increased forward elevation even in the absence of a supraspinatus tendon.[14] When repair is possible, we prefer to secure it using transosseous tunnels. If there is significant "acetabularization" of the coracoacromial arch, we try to match the humeral head replacement to the preoperative humeral head size and maintain its superiorly migrated position within the coracoacromial arch. If the greater tuberosity remains, it is smoothed to improve the congruity of the humeral head articulation with the acromion. Care should be taken to avoid overstuffing the joint with a head component that is too large, as this will result in postoperative stiffness and can lead to subscapularis failure.

The subscapularis repair is a critical part of the procedure. The subscapularis was cut as far lateral as possible to preserve its length for superior transposition to the anterior part of the greater tuberosity. The anterior repair is medialized to the cut surgical neck area of the humerus to help maximize tendon length. It is critical to have a wide bone surface on the neck of the humerus for optimum tendon-bone contact. If possible, the superior and posterior cuff should also be repaired. The posterior attachment, including the teres minor, should never be detached as this will lead to weakness of ER.

Postoperatively, rehabilitation focuses on protecting the repair of the RC repair, which in most cases is primarily the subscapularis. All patients are placed into a supervised postoperative physical therapy program for at least 6 weeks following surgery. Patients are protected in a sling for 4 to 6 weeks and they are started on pendulum exercises, ER exercises with a stick to 30 degrees, and passive supine elevation to a limit of 130 degrees. At 6 weeks, they are gradually advanced to isometrics and strengthening.

Case Study

Figure 12–6 represents an illustrative case of an 81-year-old woman with longstanding, progressive right shoulder pain and decreased active motion. Physical exam revealed active forward elevation of 90 degrees, ER of 20 degrees, and internal rotation (IR) to the side. An anteroposterior (AP) radiograph and coronal oblique magnetic resonance imaging (MRI) scan are shown in **Fig. 12–6A,B**. The patient failed nonoperative treatment including corticosteroid injection and antiinflammatory medications. She then underwent hemiarthroplasty using a Zimmer Bigliani–Flatow humeral head replacement (Zimmer, Inc., Warsaw, IN). **Fig. 12–6C–H**

depict the surgical technique and findings. She underwent rehabilitation as outlined above and achieved postoperative range of motion of 100 degrees elevation. The postoperative AP radiograph is shown in **Fig. 12–6I**.

Results

Recently, we looked up our results of hemiarthroplasty for arthritis with massive RC tears. Goldberg et al[15] reviewed 34 shoulders in 31 patients having undergone hemiarthroplasty for either CTA or osteoarthritis with a massive RC tear from 1985 to 2000. Patients with rheumatoid arthritis, osteonecrosis, or fracture sequelae were excluded. The average patient age was 72 years at surgery and the average follow-up was 8.5 (2 to 16) years. All patients underwent hemiarthroplasty with an attempted partial repair of the residual RC tissue. In all patients, both the supraspinatus and infraspinatus tendons were torn, in 35% three tendons were torn, and in 12%, four tendons were torn.

At the time of follow-up, 76% of patients had satisfied Neer's "limited goals" criteria.[5] To meet these "limited goals," the patient must have no or mild pain, must be pleased with the procedure, and must be independent with activities of daily living. There were two reoperations; an arthroscopic distal clavicle excision and a greater tuberosity exostectomy, but no revisions of the hemiarthroplasty. All patients had significant improvement in terms of forward elevation and ER. The most significant finding was that patients with preoperative active forward elevation of >90 degrees, 88% satisfied limited goals and had better pain relief ($p = 0.001$) and better ASES scores ($p = 0.002$) than those who could not actively elevate over 90 degrees preoperatively. It can be concluded that hemiarthroplasty for arthritis with a massive RC tear has good long-term results overall, low complication rates, and has excellent results in patients with preoperative active forward elevation >90 degrees.

Reverse Shoulder Arthroplasty

The shoulder is approached through a deltopectoral approach. This is chosen over the anterosuperior approach because it both preserves the deltoid and allows better visualization of the inferior glenoid, resulting in the ability to give the baseplate 10 to 15 degrees of inferior tilt. If present, the biceps tendon is released and tenodesed to soft tissues at the end of the case. The subscapularis is taken down as in the above technique for hemiarthroplasty and tagged for later repair. The humeral head is dislocated in adduction, extension, and ER. We utilize the Zimmer TM Reverse Shoulder system (Zimmer, Inc., Warsaw, IN). The humeral canal is identified and reamed to a tight fit. The reamer is then left in as an alignment guide for the humeral head cutting jig. The head is cut conservatively to maintain length and deltoid tension, with more removed later if the reduction is too

Using the Reverse Shoulder Prosthesis

From 1998 to December 2007, I had performed 773 reverse shoulder arthroplasties. We have kept a database on these patients since 1999 to promote our understanding of how this device treats the RC-deficient shoulder. We evaluate several outcome measures on each of our patients preoperatively and postoperatively and videotape each patient to assist in documenting the ROM. This has allowed us to obtain a wealth of information on this patient population.

Currently, my indications for the use of a RSP are

-Irreparable RC tear with glenohumeral arthritis
-Irreparable RC tear with glenohumeral instability
-Failed hemiarthroplasty
-Painful and loose total shoulder arthroplasty with RC deficiency

My contraindications for this surgical procedure are

-Nonfunctional deltoid muscle
-Active sepsis
-Excessive glenoid bone loss
-Debilitating neurologic disorder
-Metal allergy

Patients who meet the above indications and have failed conservative management are candidates to undergo the following surgical techniques.

Preoperative Considerations and Operative Technique

Primary Reverse Shoulder Prosthesis

All patients who undergo a primary RSP receive the same preoperative workup.[11] All patients must have recent x-rays and a preoperative computed tomography (CT) scan. The x-rays show the position of the humerus relative to the glenoid and reveal the degenerative changes of the humerus, glenoid, and acromion. The axial cuts of the CT scan are evaluated to look at the wear pattern on the glenoid and plan for proper central screw placement of the baseplate. In patients who demonstrate minimal glenoid bone loss, the ideal position of the central screw will follow the path of the centering line as described by Matsen and Lippitt[12] (**Fig. 13–3**), in which the central screw exits anteriorly on the scapular neck. This typically will provide at least 25 mm of bone for the screw to achieve purchase. In the majority of our primary RSP cases, we are able to position the central screw in this position.

For surgery, the patient is placed in the upright beach-chair position with the head firmly secured and the arm draped free. The operative arm is positioned sufficiently off the side of the table to allow for unobstructed movement in adduction and hyperextension of the shoulder (**Fig. 13–4**). The patient is administered a general anesthetic in

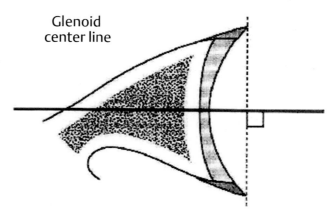

Figure 13–3 Ideal position of the central baseplate screw. This screw follows the centering line as described by Matsen.[12] The screw should exit anteriorly on the scapular neck and is typically around 25 mm in length to achieve adequate purchase.

addition to a scalene block. An extended deltopectoral approach is employed and up to two thirds of the pectoralis major tendon is released. The subdeltoid, subacromial, and subcoracoid spaces are released. If the subscapularis tendon is intact, it is released off the lesser tuberosity just medial to the long head of the biceps, allowing atraumatic dislocation of the humeral head with gentle external rotation (ER) and extension of the arm. The capsule is then released completely around the humeral neck. Aggressive

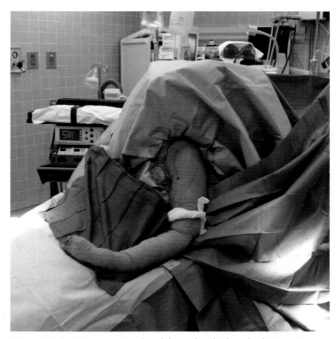

Figure 13–4 Patient prepped and draped in the beach-chair position.

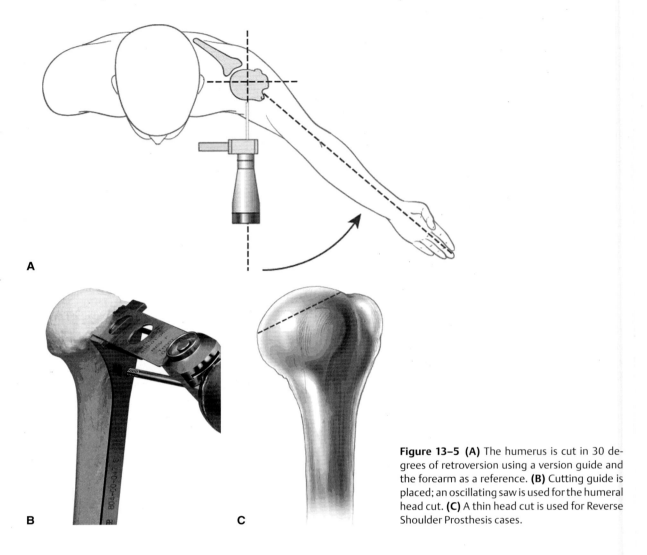

Figure 13–5 (A) The humerus is cut in 30 degrees of retroversion using a version guide and the forearm as a reference. **(B)** Cutting guide is placed; an oscillating saw is used for the humeral head cut. **(C)** A thin head cut is used for Reverse Shoulder Prosthesis cases.

resection of any osteophytes is then performed. A neck cut is made in 30 degrees of retroversion. This cut is made at a slightly higher level than for a traditional arthroplasty (**Fig. 13–5**). Sequential broaches are used to prepare the canal.

The proximal humerus is then reamed using the smallest metaphyseal reamer (**Fig. 13–6A**). Any remaining osteophytes and a portion of the calcar are then resected back to a recessed position (**Fig. 13–6B**). The humeral broach is

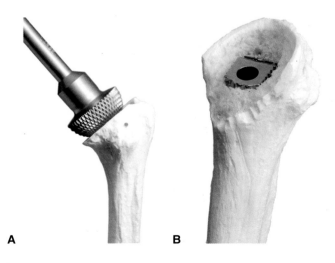

Figure 13–6 (A,B) Proximal humeral reamers are used to prepare the humerus.

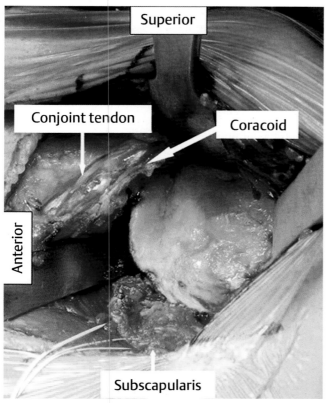

Figure 13–7 A 360-degree periglenoid exposure is performed to prepare for baseplate insertion.

left in place until implantation of the glenoid component is completed. This sequence allows for sufficient resection of the proximal humerus to aid in glenoid exposure. The delay of the last two humeral reamers until the glenoid preparation is complete maintains adequate humeral bone stock to support retraction during glenoid preparation.

Glenoid exposure is accomplished by retracting the proximal humerus posteriorly utilizing a posterior glenoid retractor, and performing an aggressive 360-degree subpe-

riosteal periglenoid capsular release. A Hohman retractor is then placed anteriorly on the glenoid neck, and a second Hohman retractor is placed at the superior aspect of the glenoid (**Fig. 13–7**). With protection of the axillary nerve, the inferior capsule is then resected. Once satisfactory visualization of the glenoid is accomplished, a centering hole is drilled using a 2.0-mm drill with a slight inferior tilt, followed by the 6.5-mm tap (**Fig. 13–8**). The tap is left in the glenoid to serve as a guide for placement of the cannulated glenoid reamers. Sequential cannulated convex reamers are then used to prepare the glenoid for the baseplate insertion (**Fig. 13–9**). Next, a fixed angle hydroxyapatite-coated glenoid baseplate is screwed into place with secure purchase (**Fig. 13–10**). Four 5.0-mm locking peripheral fixation screws are inserted into the glenoid baseplate. In cases where the locked screw pathway does not have sufficient bone, 3.5-mm nonlocking cortical screw is used and angled to achieve secure fixation in bone. An appropriately sized glenosphere (32-mm neutral, 32 - 4 mm, 36-mm neutral, 36 - 4 mm, 40-mm neutral, 40 - 4 mm) (**Fig. 13–11**) is then selected, depending on the degree of soft tissue contracture, the size of the patient, the quality of glenoid bone, and the expected degree of instability. It is placed onto the baseplate via a Morse taper. A retaining screw is then placed into the central hole on the glenosphere to augment the Morse taper attachment to the baseplate (**Fig. 13–12**). The humeral reaming is then completed and a trial humeral socket is chosen from a selection of sizes (neutral, neutral-semi-constrained, +4 mm, +4-mm semi-constrained, +8 mm, +8-mm semi-constrained) depending on the soft tissue balancing and degree of instability. After reduction with the humeral broach and a trial humeral socket (**Fig. 13–13**), transosseous sutures are placed into the lesser tuberosity for future subscapularis repair. Next, the appropriate-size humeral implant that would allow a 2-mm circumferential cement interface around the component is selected and routinely cemented in place with antibiotic-laden cement. Our standard practice has been to

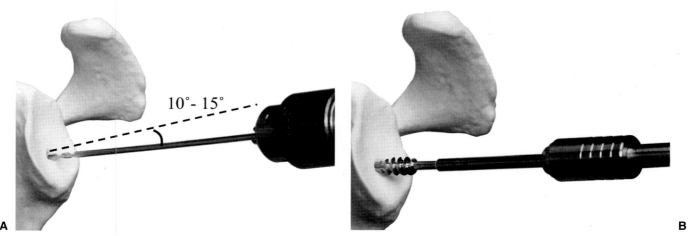

A   **B**

Figure 13–8 **(A)** A 2.5-mm drill is oriented with 10 to 15 degrees of inferior tilt. **(B)** The glenoid is tapped along the drill path.

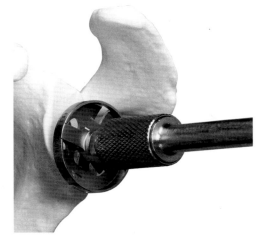

Figure 13–9 The glenoid is reamed over the tap.

use antibiotic-laden cement in all cemented arthroplasties as it has been found to reduce the risk of deep wound infection. The joint is then reduced and checked for stability especially in abduction, extension, and internal rotation (the position of greatest instability) and achievement of full passive elevation is confirmed. Finally the subscapularis is repaired through drill holes followed by routine closure using #2 braided polyester sutures. Standard radiographs are obtained immediately postoperatively (**Fig. 13–14**).

Postoperative Rehabilitation

A shoulder immobilizer is worn for 6 weeks while pendulum-type exercises are performed. After the first 6 weeks, the patient is transitioned to a sling and supine active assisted ROM exercises are initiated. Active assisted elevation can begin at 6 weeks, but resistive exercises are delayed un-

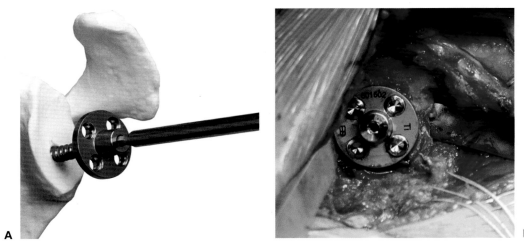

A   **B**

Figure 13–10 (A) The glenoid baseplate is then inserted. **(B)** Implanted Reverse Shoulder Prosthesis baseplate with four 5.0-mm locking screws.

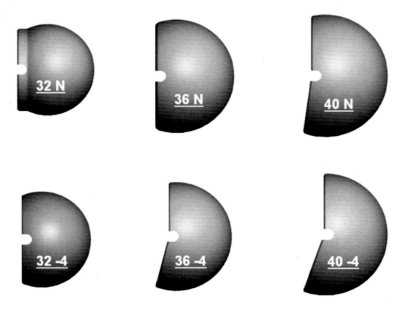

Figure 13–11 There are several options for glenosphere selection with varying diameters and offsets.

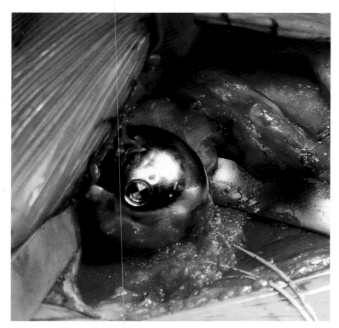

Figure 13–12 An implanted glenosphere.

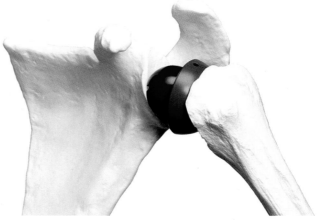

Figure 13–13 A sawbones model demonstrating a reduction with trial components in place.

til 12 weeks after surgery. Strengthening and stretching exercises should continue with maximal functional improvement expected to occur about one year after surgery.

Previous Arthroplasty and Conversion to Reverse Shoulder Prosthesis

In my practice, I encounter a high volume of referred patients who have had previous arthroplasty and remain symptomatic with a RC that is nonfunctional. These patients present with pain and poor function of the affected extremity. Their previous arthroplasties have included hemiarthroplasty or a bipolar, unconstrained total shoulder arthroplasty, and reverse shoulder arthroplasty. The etiologies for the initial arthroplasty have included proximal humeral fracture, CTA, and glenohumeral arthritis.

In these groups of revision cases, special technical measures are required. Each of these groups of patients has a specific pathology that can be due to the previous procedure they have undergone. We classify these patients into different groups based on their prior procedure because this tends to dictate the type of pathology the patient will have during revision surgery. This allows us to have a preoperative plan as to what obstacles may be encountered

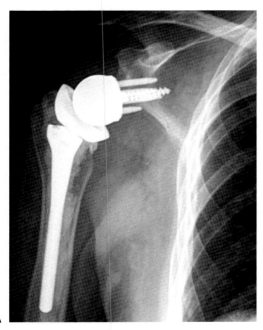

A

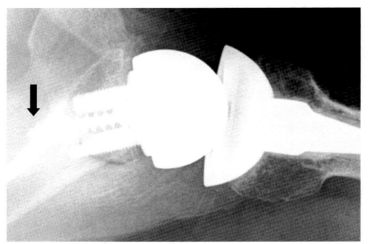

B

Figure 13–14 (A,B) Postoperative x-ray of the Reverse Shoulder Prosthesis.

during the revision and enables us to have all the necessary equipment present and ready for the case. Therefore, one must have an effective way to remove the previous implant, and then deal with the additional pathology that can be present in each of these groups of patients.

The Problems of Instability and Bone Loss

For instance, when revising a hemiarthroplasty for fracture, the surgeon should be prepared to deal with scarred down tuberosities, the proximal humeral bone loss and instability that can be present after implant removal. To optimize results, we attempt to recognize this in the preoperative setting and plan for it. Additionally, a bipolar or a hemiarthroplasty with a larger humeral head can produce a patulous deltoid, making stability an issue in attempting to convert to the RSP. In this situation, one must anticipate the need for more conforming sockets and replacing bone loss to avoid postoperative dislocation. In cases of revision after hemiarthroplasty for CTA, one must be prepared for the glenoid bone erosion that often has occurred and may require bone grafting. If it is an unconstrained total shoulder that is being converted, the surgeon should have an effective way of removing the glenoid component and cement to prepare a good bony bed for baseplate implantation. Lastly, in revising a reverse shoulder arthroplasty the surgeon must be prepared to encounter broken screws and other failed hardware. The following sections illustrate our current surgical approach of converting to the RSP in these complex cases, and have provided us with reasonable outcomes, which are described below.

Conversion Hemiarthroplasty for Fracture

The primary concern in the revision surgery of a hemiarthroplasty for fracture is removal of the implant and the potential for proximal humeral bone loss as well as instability (**Fig. 13–15**). We obtain recent plain x-rays and a CT scan of these patients prior to surgery. The plain films give us information regarding what type of humeral component is in place so we can plan for its removal, and also allows us to look at the tuberosities. The CT scan is imperative to evaluate proximal humeral bone stock as well as the position of the tuberosities because they are commonly in a malunited or nonunited position. If the CT scan reveals a greater tuberosity that has retracted to a posterior position, it is valuable information in that we will have to look for this fragment at the time of surgery. Failure to remove this fragment at the time surgery can influence the patient outcome and cause pain, a decrease in postoperative ROM, or possible instability. The CT scan also provides detail of the glenoid anatomy to plan for the central screw placement of our baseplate. Before these cases, we are sure to

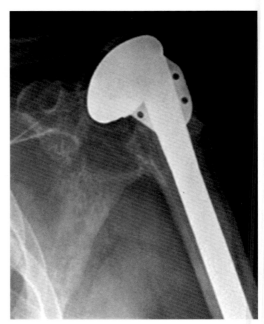

Figure 13–15 Failed hemiarthroplasty with proximal humeral bone loss, superior migration of the humeral component, and glenoid erosion.

request a proximal humeral allograft as this may be required during surgery.

For surgery the patient is positioned in the upright beach-chair position and is administered a general anesthetic in addition to a scalene block. The skin incision may utilize previous skin incisions if they are close to the deltopectoral interval. If the previous incision is not in close proximity to the deltopectoral groove a separate skin incision must be made. This incision is centered directly over the deltopectoral groove and is often longer than the incision used for primary surgery. By making the incision slightly longer, it allows for identification of undisturbed tissue planes and can assist in defining normal anatomical planes.

Meticulous dissection must be done using a layered approach; it often takes additional time due to thick scar formation. Large subcutaneous flaps are created to correctly identify the deltoid and the pectoralis major. Once the correct location of the deltopectoral interval is found, it can then be divided. First, the deltoid needs to be identified and adequately mobilized. We try to begin proximally, as described above, and find the triangular fat interval between the proximal deltoid and pectoralis major. If this plane has become obscured due to scar tissue, we start distally separating the distal deltoid from the humeral shaft and then working proximally. The use of Homan retractors placed under the proximal deltoid and under the acromion may help to develop the subdeltoid and subacromial spaces, which must be freed. Often the pectoralis major may be scarred down to the conjoined tendon. Additional time is taken to identify the pectoralis major and separate it from the underlying conjoined tendon. Separating these two structures is necessary to find the lateral edge of the conjoined tendon.

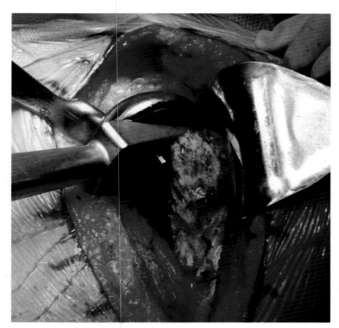

Figure 13–16 Intraoperative photo showing removal of the head component.

Once this is found, the subcoracoid space can be identified and freed from the underlying subscapularis, which can be scarred to the conjoined tendon. The axillary nerve can then be palpated, and a tug test is performed.

Next, the RC is assessed to identify remaining portions. If the subscapularis tendon is intact, it is released subperiosteally from the proximal humerus, allowing atraumatic dislocation of the humeral hemiarthroplasty with gentle ER and extension of the arm. The humeral capsule is released circumferentially from the humeral neck. If the humeral prosthesis is modular, the humeral head is dislodged from the Morse taper of the humeral stem using a forked wedge impactor (**Fig. 13–16**). The tuberosity position and integrity are then assessed. If either tuberosity is malunited, it is removed to freely release the RC. Additionally, if the greater tuberosity is healed in an inferoposterior position the RC is released off this fragment.

Removal of the hemiarthroplasty is performed in a stepwise fashion. Circumferential exposure of the proximal portion of the humeral component is established with the removal of all soft tissue, bone ingrowth, and cement from around the humeral head, collar, and fins of the prosthesis. This is accomplished using careful dissection with the aid of an osteotome and a high speed burr. In cases of proximally coated stems, a thin flexible osteotome is used to create space between the prosthesis and the bone or cement interface (**Fig. 13–17**). Once the medial neck and fins are properly exposed (**Fig. 13–18**), the arm is elevated to 90 degrees of abduction and placed on a Mayo stand. The Carbide punch bone tamp (Moreland Revision Set; DePuy Orthopaedics, Inc., Warsaw, Indiana) is placed onto an edge on the medial neck of the prosthesis, and a mallet is used to deliver a series of controlled horizontal forehand blows parallel to the humeral shaft to initially dislodge the hemiarthroplasty from the cortical bone or cement mantle (**Fig. 13–19**). Once the prosthesis is loose, the arm is placed into full adduction and the tamp is used in an upward fashion parallel to the humeral shaft to deliver the hemiarthroplasty stem out of the intramedullary canal (**Fig. 13–20**). In cases in which the stem is difficult to remove, more aggressive measures may have to be taken to loosen the implant. In these cases the humerus can be split along the medial cortex to facilitate stem removal (**Fig. 13–21**). If that is unsuccessful, a larger medial window can be created to dislodge the stem and remove the implant (**Fig. 13–22**).

Once the humeral hemiarthroplasty is removed, the subscapularis is tagged for future repair. Any additional heterotopic ossification and osteophytes are resected. When present, the previous cement mantle is left intact. Sequential handheld diaphyseal reamers are placed within

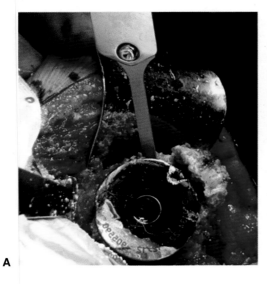

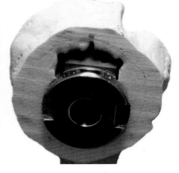

A

B

Figure 13–17 (A) Intraoperative photo demonstrating use of a flexible osteotome to expose all fins of the humeral implant. **(B)** Sawbones model demonstrating humeral component prior to exposure of fins.

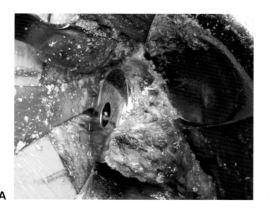

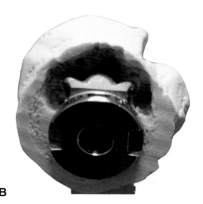

Figure 13–18 (A) Intraoperative photo showing exposure fins on the humeral component. **(B)** Sawbones model showing fins now exposed.

the intramedullary canal to gently prepare the humerus, and a trial broach is introduced until it is seated just distal to the neck cut. The remainder of the surgical procedure consists of inserting the RSP in a similar manner to that described earlier in this chapter. The main difference in these cases of conversion of the hemiarthroplasty for fracture is that a proximal humeral allograft may need to be added due to humeral bone loss. In our early revision arthroplasty cases, we have experienced some polyethylene failures in patients who had moderate to severe bone loss preoperatively on the humeral side and did not have a proximal humeral allograft placed.

In cases where the proximal humerus has severe bone loss (**Fig. 13–23**), we now employ the use of a proximal humeral allograft to support the cemented humeral component. A fresh frozen humeral allograft is prepared to match the proximal humerus. To do this, we cut the humeral head of the proximal humeral allograft at the level of the anatomical neck and remove all the cancellous allograft bone from the intramedullary canal. We then determine the appropriate height of the allograft by inspecting how much diaphyseal bone remains and estimating how much proximal humerus will need to be replaced to restore the bone stock and allow for a stable reduction (**Fig. 13–24**). An os-

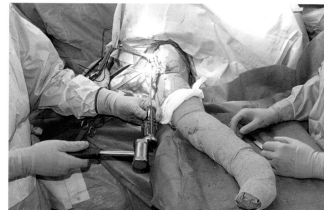

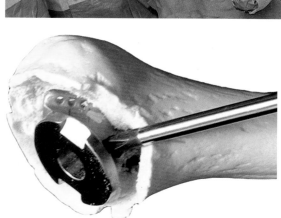

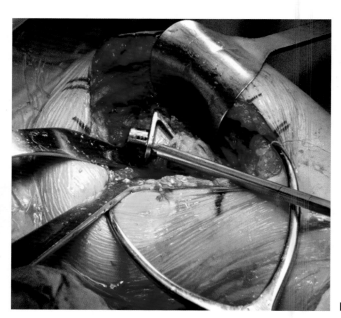

Figure 13–19 (A) The arm is initially placed in 90 degrees of abduction on a Mayo stand to allow the surgeon to use parallel forehand blows in line with the humerus in an effort to loosen the prosthesis. **(B,C)** A tamp is placed on the medial aspect of the prosthesis as the forehand blows are applied.

were compared.[14] The group without surgery showed an average improvement from 15.0 to 39.8 ($p < 0.0001$), and the group with previous surgery improved from 16.1 to 37.6 ($p < 0.0001$). Both groups have shown statistically significant improvements with respect to preoperative and postoperative ASES functional scores. The group without surgery showed average improvements of 15.9 to 30.6 ($p < 0.0001$), and the previous surgery group improved from 16.2 to 28.8 ($p < 0.0001$). The visual analog scores for function and pain also showed statistically significant improvements postoperatively.

With respect to ROM, each group of patients has had statistically significant improvements in their forward elevation and abduction. The patients without surgery improved their forward elevation from 61 to 122 degrees ($p < 0.0001$) and their abduction from 50 to 111 degrees ($p < 0.0001$). When considering ER, the group of patients without surgery demonstrated an average postoperative increase of 12 degrees ($p < 0.005$). The group with prior surgery showed a slight increase in postoperative ER, but did not reach statistical significance. Overall, treatment of the RC-deficient shoulder with the RSP has been a very reliable way to decrease our patients' pain and improve their function.

Conversion of Failed Hemiarthroplasty for Fracture to the Reverse Shoulder Prosthesis

Some of the techniques mentioned here grew out of our experience with patients who have had a failed hemiarthroplasty for fracture. These patients may present with stiffness, tuberosity malunion, or nonunion resulting in a nonfunctional RC, instability, and glenoid arthritis. These failures related to glenoid arthritis and RC deficiency due to tuberosity malunion, nonunion, or resorption can be devastating to the patient's function. Since 2007, we have had 61 patients who were treated for failed hemiarthroplasty for fracture with conversion to the RSP and are at least 2 years into their follow-up. Of this group, 5 have passed away and 2 have been lost to follow-up, leaving 54 shoulders available for our analysis. All of these patients had some degree of glenoid arthritis and an irreparable RC due to malunion, nonunion, or tuberosity resorption. All of these patients were managed with a single-stage conversion. Of this group of patients, some were treated with a proximal humeral allograft in conjunction with the implantation of the RSP.

These patients had a substantial improvement in their pain and functional scores. The ASES scores for pain improved from 13.2 to 31.8 ($p < 0.0001$) and the ASES function scores improved for 13.0 to 19.4 ($p = 0.015$). The visual analog scores for pain and function also showed statistically significant improvements. The forward flexion in this group of patients went from 45.7 to 74.2 degrees after surgery ($p = 0.0002$). Abduction improved from 36.6 to 66.4 degrees after surgery ($p < 0.0001$).

This group of patients presents a difficult predicament for the shoulder surgeon. The addition of the proximal humeral allograft has become an important component of our reconstruction on the humeral side in these cases. Given our experiences we feel that this procedure is a viable salvage for patients who have a failed hemiarthroplasty for fracture and have no other reconstruction options. The surgery is technically demanding and can have significant complications.

Failed Hemiarthroplasty for Glenoid Arthritis and a Rotator Cuff-Deficient Shoulder

We have followed a group of patients who had severe pain and loss of function after undergoing an index procedure of hemiarthroplasty for glenohumeral arthritis associated with severe RC deficiency. It is in this patient population that we most consistently encounter some degree of glenoid bone. Over time, the hemiarthroplasty tends to migrate proximally and erode the articular surface of the glenoid, producing pain. It is not uncommon for us to be required to perform our glenoid bone-grafting techniques in these cases due to significant glenoid bone loss. To date, we have 20 shoulders in 19 patients whom we have followed for >2 years after we performed their revision surgery. Each of these patients was treated with a single-stage conversion to a RSP. The average age at the time of revision surgery was 72 years old.

We have performed preoperative and postoperative clinical and radiographic assessments on these patients. We felt it was important to document the position of the arthroplasty with respect to subluxation, and to radiographically evaluate the amount of bone loss on the glenoid and humeral sides before and after conversion to the RSP. We noted that 90% of the shoulders (18/20) had moderate to severe static shift in joint position preoperatively. Moderate to severe peripheral glenoid erosion was seen in 65% (13/20), and 40% (8/20) had moderate to severe acromial erosion.

Clinically, the results from this group of patients have been promising. All patients had statistically significant improvements in their visual analog scale pain score and functional score. Statistically significant improvements were also seen in the average total ASES scores, forward flexion (49.7 to 76.1 degrees), and abduction (42.2 to 77.2 degrees).

The goal of the conversion to the RSP in this group of patients was pain relief, and was achieved in all the patients. It was an added bonus that we found statistically significant improvements in functional scores and ROM. In our experience, conversion to the RSP is a good option to treat the patient with a failed hemiarthroplasty who has significant pain and poor function.

Failed Total Shoulder Arthroplasty Converted to the Reverse Shoulder Prosthesis

Conventional unconstrained total shoulder arthroplasty requires a functional RC for the shoulder to perform properly. We have performed revision surgery in a group of patients who had a primary total shoulder arthroplasty in which the RC has subsequently failed. These patients presented with pain and decreased function due to the proximal migration of the humeral component. To date, we have 17 shoulders which underwent this conversion and are at least 2 years out from their revision surgery. Two patients have passed away leaving 15 for analysis with at least 2 years of follow-up.

Our results in this group show that conversion to the RSP can decrease pain and increase function. These patients' ASES pain scores went from 18.3 to 33.1 ($p = 0.0062$) and the ASES functional scores improved from 11.6 to 25.4 ($p = 0.0022$) after surgery. The visual analog pain scores decreased ($p = 0.0062$) and the visual analog function scores increased ($p = .0003$). The average preoperative forward flexion for these patients was 36 degrees and increased to 93 degrees after surgery ($p = 0.0005$). The abduction went from 29 to 83 degrees ($p = 0.0004$) and ER improved from 8 to 51 degrees ($p = 0.0073$).

Conversion of Bipolar Arthroplasty

To date we have converted 11 bipolar arthroplasties to the RSP. Nine of these have follow-up greater than 2 years and are available for analysis. Due to the small sample size, we have not been able to achieve statistical significance with respect to patient outcomes, despite the fact the trends demonstrate improvement postoperatively. The data we have shows postoperative improvement in ASES pain and function scores, visual analog pain and function scores, and ROM.

Revision of Reverse Prosthesis and Conversion to the Reverse Shoulder Prosthesis

To date, we have revised 16 reverse shoulder arthroplasties and converted them to the RSP, nine of whom have greater than 2-year follow-up and are available for analysis. This group of patients have demonstrated improvement in their ASES scores from 33.1 to 71.9 ($p = 0.0089$). They have also had statistically significant improvement in forward flexion from 63 to 134 degrees ($p = 0.001$) and abduction from 45 to 107 degrees ($p = 0.0004$).

Complications

The Reverse Shoulder Replacement has been associated with certain complications. Some of these complications have been related to the prosthesis itself, whereas others were related to the pathology that was treated. We have experienced complications on the glenoid and humeral side of the arthroplasty, and have also dealt with issues of acromial fracture, component disassociation, instability, and infection. Complications are much more common in the revision setting because these are technically more difficult operations. Revision surgery with the RSP in our studies showed a high complication rate (30%). This is similar to other large series in the literature. Boileau et al[14] reported 42% of his patients required reoperation after conversion of failed hemiarthroplasty to a reverse prosthesis. Based on our experience the high complication rate in revision surgery appears to be related to the amount of preoperative bone loss. As noted earlier in the chapter, over the years we have made modifications to the device and to our techniques in an effort to minimize these complications.

The main glenoid complication we have encountered has been due to failure of fixation of the baseplate. In designing an implant with a more lateral COR, the forces at the glenoid are increased in comparison to the more medial COR in Grammont's design. In our early series, almost all the failures requiring revision were due to mechanical failure of the baseplate. In each of the revision surgeries, evaluation of the porous surface of the glenoid baseplate revealed no evidence of osseous ingrowth. The number of glenoid baseplate failures in this initial study prompted us to explore ways to improve the baseplate fixation. Since our initial study, we have made the previously mentioned changes to our technique, most notably using 5.0-mm locked cortical screws to secure the baseplate. Prior to making this change we had a total of 23 baseplate failures. Since making this change, we have seen a marked improvement in our fixation and have had zero baseplate failures. We will continue to follow this cohort of patients closely and plan to report these findings at their 2-year postoperative point. In the revision setting our glenoid complications have been much higher in the patients with significant bone loss. Our positioning of our central screw in dense bone, and the glenosphere option of a more medial COR have helped to limit glenoid complications in the patients with poor bone stock.

On the humeral side, we have treated four postoperative periprosthetic fractures. These have been related to patient falls or trauma. A few of these patients have required revision surgery with either open reduction and fixation or conversion to a long-stem prosthesis. We have also seen polyethelene failure on the humeral side in a third of our patients. These were patients in our revision of hemiarthroplasty group who had experienced proximal humeral bone loss and were not treated with a proximal humeral allograft at the time of their revision. In our series on failed hemiarthroplasty the patients who did undergo proximal humeral allograft did not encounter this problem. We believe the cortical support of the allograft provides additional rotational and structural stability, thereby decreasing stress on the humeral component. We now employ the use of proximal humeral allografting in our patients with severe bone loss. In our series of primary reverse shoulder arthroplasty, we have seen only one case of humeral loosening and this has not been a significant issue.

Instability is another complication seen in our patients after undergoing reversed arthroplasty. We have had an overall dislocation rate of 3.1% (24/773). Two modifications have been used to improve the stability of the glenohumeral articulation. Larger glenospheres (36 mm and 40 mm) are now available and used. This allows for greater coverage than the smaller diameter 32 mm head. Deeper, semi-constrained sockets are available for the humeral side to provide greater stability at the articulation if instability is a concern.

Component disassociation has been a reported complication of reversed arthroplasty. Humeral disassociation has occurred in 1.2% (9/773) of our patients and glenosphere disassociation has occurred in 0.5% (4/773). To combat this, we have added a 3.5-mm retaining screw to lock the glenosphere to the baseplate and augment the Morse taper between the two components. Additionally, a metal shell has been added to the polyethylene liner on the humeral socket to limit this complication.

Acromial fracture has been reported in the literature and has been seen in our patient population. Overall we have had four patients sustain a postoperative acromial fracture. One of these acromial fractures was felt to be a result of overaggressive physical therapy. Consequently, we no longer use a formal physical therapist in the early postoperative setting. Patients are instructed how to do active assisted ROM at the 6-week point and do these exercises themselves. At present, patients who sustain an acromial fracture are treated symptomatically and open reduction and internal fixation is not performed.

Deep postoperative infections have occurred in 2.1% (16/773) of our patients. These have been treated with aggressive débridements, intravenous antibiotics, and retention of the prosthesis. We have not had to remove any implants for recurrent infections that were not able to be eradicated. In our series, there have been three cases of postoperative hematoma that required return to the operating room for evacuation of the hematoma.

It is important to note that scapular notching is a common reported complication of those patients treated with a reversed device that has the COR at the glenoid. In a recent multicenter study using this type of device, the incidence of notching was reported at 64%.[17] In our series of patients treated with the RSP with the more lateral offset of the COR, scapular notching has not been an issue. We feel this is one of the significant benefits to this design.

Conclusion

The development of the RSP has been an interesting journey. In our attempts to find a better way to treat patients, we have gained significant insight into the RC-deficient shoulder. We have utilized clinical data, biomechanical studies, and implant design to arrive at a treatment that we feel is the best option to help these patients now. In the coming years, we will continue to follow our patients closely in an effort to continue to gain more information about the RC-deficient shoulder and the RSP.

References

1. Parsons IM, Apreleva M, Fu FJ et al. The effect of rotator cuff tears on reaction forces at the glenohumeral joint. J Orthop Res 2002; 20(3):439–446
2. Cofield RH, Briggs BT. Glenohumeral arthrodesis. Operative and long-term functional results. J Bone Joint Surg Am 1979;61(5):668–677
3. Lettin AW, Copelan SA, Scales JT. The Stanmore total shoulder replacement. J Bone Joint Surg Br 1982;64(1):47–51
4. Franklin JL, Barrett WP, Jackine SE, et al. Glenoid loosening in total shoulder arthroplasty. Association with rotator cuff deficiency. J Arthroplasty 1988;3(1):39–46
5. Arntz CT, Matsen RA III, Jackins S. Surgical management of complex irreparable rotator cuff deficiency. J Arthroplasty 1991;6(4):363–370
6. Sanchez-Sotelo J, Cofield RH, Rowland CM. Shoulder hemiarthroplasty for glenohumeral arthritis associated with severe rotator cuff deficiency. J Bone Joint Surg Am 2001;83-A(12):1814–1822
7. Fenlin JM Jr. Total glenohumeral joint replacement. Orthop Clin North Am 1975;6(2):565–583
8. Grammont PM, Baulot E. Delta shoulder prosthesis for rotator cuff rupture. Orthopedics 1993;16(1):65–68
9. Jacobs R, Debeer P, De Smet L. Treatment of rotator cuff arthropathy with reversed Delta shoulder prosthesis. Acta Orthop Belg 2001;67(4):344–347
10. Boulahia A, Edwards TB, Walch G, et al. Early results of a reverse design prosthesis in the treatment of arthritis of the shoulder in elderly patients with a large rotator cuff tear. Orthopedics 2002;25(2):129–133
11. Frankle M, Levy J, Pupello D, Siegal S, Saleem A, Mighell M, Vasey M. The reverse shoulder prosthesis for glenohumeral arthritis associated with severe rotator cuff deficiency. A minimum two-year follow-up study of sixty patients: Surgical technique. JBJS Am Sep 2006;88:178–190
12. Matsen MA, Lippitt SB. Shoulder Surgery Principles and Procedures. 1st ed. Philadelphia, PA: WB Saunders; 2004:495–496
13. Harman M, Frankle M, Vasey M, Banks S. Initial glenoid component fixation in reverse total shoulder arthroplasty: a biomechanical evaluation. J Shoulder Elbow Surg 2005; 14(1): S162–S167

14. Richards RR, An KN, Bigliani LU, Friedman RJ, Gartsman GM, Gristina AG, et al. A standardized method for the assessment of shoulder function. J Shoulder Elbow Surg 1994;3:347–352

15. Gutierrez S, Griewe M, Frankle M, Siegal S. Biomechanical comparison of component position and hardware failure in the reverse shoulder prosthesis. J Shoulder Elbow Surg 2007;35:9–12

16. Boileau P, Watkinson DJ, Hatzidakis AM, Balg F. Grammont reverse prosthesis: design, rational, and biomechanics. J Shoulder Elbow Surg 2005;14:147s–161s

17. Sirveaux F, Favard L, Oudet D, Huquet D, Walch G, Mole D. Grammont inverted total shoulder arthroplasty in the treatment of glenohumeral osteoarthritis with massive rupture of the cuff. Results of a multicentre study of 80 shoulders. J Bone Joint Surg Br 2004;86:388–395

18. Williams GR Jr, Rockwood CA Jr. Hemiarthroplasty in rotator cuff-deficient shoulders. J Shoulder Elbow Surg 1996;5(5):362–367

19. Pollock RG, Deliz ED, McIlveen SJ, et al. Prosthetic replacement in rotator cuff deficient shoulders. Orthopaedic Transactions 1993;16:774–775

14 Tissue Engineering for the Rotator Cuff–Deficient Shoulder

Joshua S. Dines, Daniel P. Grande, and David M. Dines

Surgical repair of rotator cuff (RC) tears often results in good to excellent results. However, when evaluated by ultrasound or magnetic resonance imaging (MRI), up to 50% of these tears has been shown to fail to heal.[1-6] Many patients improve clinically; nevertheless, results are clearly better in cases where the repaired tendon heals.[1,2] Initially, efforts to enhance healing focused on improving mechanical factors, such as the type of suture used, type of knots used, and anchor configuration. Recently, studies have focused on improving the biologic process of healing.[7-10] Extracellular matrix scaffolds, growth factors, and gene therapy all may play a role in improving RC tendon healing in the future. In addition, the ideal healing of massive RC tears will involve reversal of the fatty muscle degeneration that accompanies these tears.

Extracellular Matrix Scaffolds

At this time, extracellular matrices (ECMs) are the most commonly used biologic augments to tendon healing. ECMs are commercially available patches that are Food & Drug Administration (FDA) approved for clinical use for reinforcement of soft tissues that are repaired with suture or suture anchors during RC surgery.[3] The scaffolds provide a three-dimensional matrix, which can attract host cells and can provide a site-specific matrix for cell migration. They are resorbable materials around which the body rebuilds more structurally and functionally appropriate treatment. Dejardin's study,[4] in which porcine small intestine submucosa (SIS; DePuy Biologics, Raynham, Massachusetts) was used to treat RC tears in dogs, showed that eventually the patch is reabsorbed from the implantation site; and it is re-placed with site-appropriate, host-derived tissue. Because these ECMs are not approved as interposition material to replace absent tendon or to provide the full mechanical strength for the tendon repair, they tend to offer more of a biologic than mechanical advantage with regards to tendon healing. The two main groups of ECMs are those from dermis and those from small intestine submucosa (**Table 14-1**).

Collagen-rich ECMs from small intestine submucosa (SIS) include the Restore Patch and the CuffPatch.[5] The Restore Patch (Depuy Orthopaedics, Warsaw Indiana) was the first ECM to receive FDA approval for use in RC repair. It is comprised of 10 layers of porcine small intestine submucosa that has been devitalized so that it theoretically does not contain any viable cells. That being said, a recent study actually confirmed the presence of porcine DNA in Restore.[6] It is likely that this is a remnant of tissue processing. The extracellular matrix of the SIS is comprised mainly of type I collagen, fibronectin, chondroitin sulfate, heparin sulfate, and a variety of growth factors, including transforming growth factor-beta (TGF-β), vascular endothelial growth factor (VEGF), and fibroblast growth factor 2 (FGF-2).[9-15] Restore is not artificially cross-linked, and it is packaged in a dehydrated form. This contrasts with the CuffPatch (Arthrotek, Warsaw Indiana), which is an eight-layer, acellular, porcine SIS scaffold. Unlike the Restore, following lamination of the layers, the ECM is cross-linked, and it is packaged in its hydrated form.

GraftJacket, TissueMend, Zimmer Collagen Repair Patch, and Permacol are ECMs derived from dermis.[7] GraftJacket Regenerative Tissue Matrix (Wright Medical, Arlington, Texas) comes from processed human allograft skin from which the epidermis, cells, and cell remnants have been re-

Table 14-1 Commercially Available Extracellular Matrices Patches for Rotator Cuff Repair

Product	Manufacturer	Source	Tissue type	Chemically cross-linked?
GraftJacket tissue matrix	Wright medical (Arlington, Tennessee)	Human	Dermis	No
TissueMend soft tissue repair matrix	Stryker Orthopaedics (Mahwah, New Jersey)	Bovine	Fetal dermis	No
Zimmer collagen repair patch	Zimmer (Warsaw, Indiana)	Porcine	Dermis	Yes
Restore orthobiologic implant	DePuy Orthopaedics (Warsaw, Indiana)	Porcine	Small intestine submucosa (SIS)	No
CuffPatch bioengineered tissue reinforcement	Arthrotek (Warsaw, Indiana)	Porcine	Small intestine submucosa (SIS)	Yes

From Derwin K, Baker A, Spragg K, Leigh D, Iannotti JP. Commercial extracellular matrix scaffolds for rotator cuff tendon repair: biomechanical, biochemical, and cellular properties. J Bone Joint Surg Am 2006; 88:2265–2272. Adapted by permission

moved. The remaining dermal layer is freeze dried to retain the extracellular architecture and vascular channels.[7] Biochemical components in the matrix include collagen, elastin, and proteoglycans. Like the Restore patch, it is packaged dry and is not cross-linked. The patch comes in a variety of thicknesses, which can be used for different surgical situations.

TissueMend Soft Tissue Repair matrix (Stryker Orthopaedics, Mahwah, New Jersey) is derived from fetal bovine dermis.[7] It is an acellular, non-artificially cross-linked collagen membrane that is one layer thick. Type I and type III collagens are the primary component of the ECM. TissueMend is packaged dry.

The Zimmer Collagen Repair Patch (Zimmer, Warsaw, Indiana) is very similar to the Permacol surgical implant.[7] Both are acellular sheets of cross-linked porcine dermis. Cellular material, fats, and soluble proteins are removed prior to the material being cross-linked with diisocyanate, which makes it resistant to enzymatic degradation.

Derwin and colleagues performed an in vitro study comparing the biochemical, biomechanical, and cellular properties of these patches to each other and to normal tendon.[7] Samples of GraftJacket, TissueMend, Restore, and CuffPatch were tested for stiffness and modulus. In addition, hydroxyproline, glycosaminoglycan, and DNA content were quantified. The group found that commercial ECMs required 10 to 30% stretch before the patches started to bear significant load. Once stretched enough, though, each ECM exhibited a stiffer, linear region and an appreciable breaking strength.[7] Overall, SIS ECMs (Restore, Cuffpatch) were stiffer than those of dermal origin (GraftJacket, TissueMend) and reached their maximum mechanical properties at lower levels of stretch. At physiological levels of strain for tendon, the biomechanically tested, material properties of the ECMs tested were an order of magnitude less than human RC tendon (**Fig. 14–1**). In terms of biochemical composition, the ECMs tested had similar amounts of hydroxyproline and chondroitin/dermatan sulfate glycosaminoglycan as fresh tendon.[7] Despite being

marketed as "acellularized" biomaterials, TissueMend, Restore, and Graftjacket all contained measurable amounts of DNA; only in CuffPatch was DNA content negligible.

The results of this study support the argument that these patches tend to be more of a biological enhancement to healing as opposed to devices intended to restore mechanical function. Because there are limited clinical studies evaluating the use of ECMs in RC repair, it is difficult to comment on the implications of animal DNA in these patches. Acellularization is performed for three reasons: to reduce antigenicity,[8] enhance host cell infiltration with appropriate cells,[9] and prevent transmission of infection.[12] Case reports of noninfectious edema, following the use of Restore, contend that the reactions are, in part, due to the presence of porcine DNA. However, further studies are needed to determine the clinical implications of incomplete acellularization.[13,14] To date, only a few clinical studies evaluate ECMs for RC repair.

Clinical Studies of Extracellular Matrices

Small intestine submucosa ECMs have been used successfully in the repair of abdominal walls,[13] vascular grafts,[14] and bladder reconstruction.[15] The orthopedic literature has several studies documenting the enhancement of tendon healing secondary to the use of SIS scaffolds.[16–24] Unfortunately, clinical studies have not been as promising. Sclamberg et al[19] retrospectively reviewed 11 consecutive patients who underwent open treatment with SIS reinforcement for massive or large RC tears. Patients were evaluated with postoperative MRI at a minimum of 6 months after the index repair and with clinical exam. Re-tears were documented in 10 of 11 patients. Only one repair remained intact per MRI at 10 months postoperatively. There were no statistically significant differences between preoperative and postoperative shoulder scores, and 5 patients scored worse postoperatively. The authors

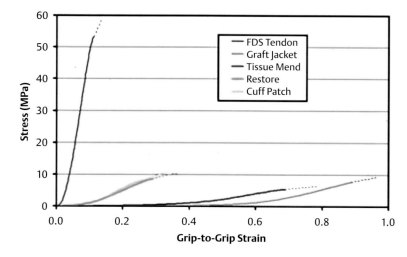

Figure 14–1 Stress-strain curves of FDS Tendon compared with extracellular matrices. (From Derwin K, Baker A, Spragg K, Leigh D, Iannotti JP. Commercial extracellular matrix scaffolds for rotator cuff tendon repair: biomechanical, biochemical, and cellular properties. J Bone Joint Surg Am 2006; 88:2265–2272. Reprinted by permission.)

concluded that the use of SIS ECMs for large and massive RC tears is ineffective.

A more recent study by Iannotti et al[13] echoed these poor results. A randomized, controlled study was performed on 30 patients with large or massive, chronic two-tendon tears. The RCs were treated with open repair using bone tunnels and a combination of modified Mason–Allen and horizontal sutures; and all patients underwent concomitant acromioplasty. Fifteen patients were randomized to a group that underwent repair augmented with the Restore patch. The patch was sewn under tension over the top of the repair from tendon to bone. All patients were evaluated at one year postoperatively with magnetic resonance arthrogram (MRA), PENN shoulder score, and SF-36 questionnaire. Nine of 15 repairs healed in the control group versus four in the augmented group ($p = 0.11$). When the rate of healing was adjusted for the effect of tear size, repairs done without the Restore patch were 7% more likely to heal. In addition, the median postoperative PENN shoulder score was 83 points in the augmented repair group and 91 in the control group. In this study, 15 more patients would have been needed to show a statistically significant less favorable result with the use of the Restore patch; however, according to the authors, ". . . there was no reason to continue the protocol . . . when [they] already had a clear indication that augmentation would not improve the clinical result."[13] The authors concluded that surgical repair with SIS did not improve the rate of tendon healing and did not improve clinical outcome scores. In fact, there was a trend toward less favorable results in patients treated with the ECM.[13]

The use of these scaffolds is not without complications. In the above referenced study by Iannotti et al, 3 of the 15 patients developed a sterile inflammatory reaction. These manifestations developed between 3 and 4 weeks postoperatively. One patient was treated with irrigation and débridement; one was treated with oral antibiotics until results from a shoulder aspiration came back as negative for infection; and the final patient's symptoms (erythema and increased skin temperature) resolved without treatment. The final PENN shoulder scores in these patients tended to be among the highest for the augmentation group, indicating that these reactions did effect final outcome.[13] Malcarney and colleagues reported on 25 patients undergoing RC repair with a Restore patch augment.[14] Four of these patients developed an overt inflammatory reaction at an average of 13 days after surgery. All patients were treated with open irrigation and débridement. As mentioned above, it is possible that these reactions stem from porcine DNA still present in the patch, but further immunologic studies and increased clinical follow up is necessary to better understand the potential complications of these ECMs.

The use of ECMs in animal models has produced good results in terms of improved healing. Unfortunately, these results have not extrapolated well to human beings, especially when used for large or massive tears. In the future, as our understanding of these scaffolds and tissue engineering improves, we may be able to modify these ECMs with growth factors to enhance their biological effects and with other materials to enhance their mechanical contribution. Preclinical studies are already underway using different growth factors to enhance RC tendon healing.

Biologic Process of Tendon Healing

Over the past 5 years, our knowledge of the healing process of RC tears and the growth factors involved has increased tremendously. Tendon architecture consists of collagen fibrils embedded in a matrix of proteoglycan.[20] Type I collagen predominates, and between the collagen bundles are fibroblasts (the most prevalent cell type in tendons).[21] During the first week of tendon healing, proliferating tissue from the paratendon penetrates the gap between the tendon stumps and fills the gap with undifferentiated, disorganized fibroblasts. Capillary buds invade the area and with the fibroblasts, compose the granulation tissue between the tendon ends. By day 3, collagen synthesis can be detected; after about 2 weeks, the tendon ends appear to be fused by a fibrous bridge. Fibroblast proliferation and collagen production in the granulation tissue continues, and between the third and fourth weeks, the fibroblasts begin to orient themselves along the axis of the tendon. Collagen fibers at the site of the tear initially remain disorganized, while collagen distant to the lesion becomes more organized.[22]

Many recent studies have focused on the intrinsic healing properties of RC tendons.[3,4,7–13] Kobayashi et al[3] showed that in the healing of full-thickness tears of avian supracoracoid tendon, the expression of $\alpha 1$ (III) lasted longer than $\alpha 1$ (I) procollagen messenger ribonucleic acid (mRNA). Studies overwhelmingly support the belief that the healing process progresses from the bursal side to the joint side.[23,24] This was shown in an experimentally created, full-thickness tear of the RC tendon.[9] In a rat model study, it was noted that type XII collagen, aggrecan, and biglycan were also increased in the healing tissue.[3] Type XII collagen is a fibril-associated collagen that binds to type-I collagen and projects into the ground matrix. Based on a study of acute supraspinatus tendon tears in a rabbit model that showed an inhibition of the healing process by matrix metalloproteinase (MMP-2), tissue inhibitor matrix metalloproteinase 1 (TIMP-1; an inhibitor of the MMP family) was used to enhance healing.[25] Another interesting finding was that a large percentage of fibroblasts in the torn, human RC contain smooth muscle actin (SMA).[8]

Several different growth factors have been studied for their effects on tendon cells, such as TGF-β, growth differentiation factor 5 (GDF-5) platelet-derived growth factor-β (PDGF-β), and insulin-like growth factor-1 (IGF-1). TGF-β increases the level of SMA, and hence fibroblasts in these tissues. Myofibroblasts have been thought to play a role in wound contracture and the retractile phenomenon observed during the fibrotic process.[26] GDF-5, a member of the TGF-β superfamily, has been shown to enhance tendon healing in animal models. A study by Nakase et al showed that cartilage-derived morphogenic protein 1 (CDMP1; an analogue of GDF-5) is activated at the site of RC tendon tears.[27,28] Yoshikawa and Abrahamsson[29] studied the effects of PDGF-β on proteoglycan, collagen, noncollagen protein, and DNA synthesis in tendons during short-term cultures. PDGF-β stimulated DNA and matrix synthesis in a dose-dependent manner in multiple tendon types IGF-1 is another growth factor with possible clinical utility in tendon repair.[30] Intratendinous injection of IGF-1 was delivered to an equine flexor tendonitis model. At the conclusion of the study, harvested tendons that received IGF-1 exhibited decreased local soft tissue swelling. In addition, cell proliferation and collagen content was increased compared with the controls. Biomechanically, the IGF-1-treated tendons were stiffer. This data supports the potential use of locally administered IGF-1 to affect tendon healing. Clearly, many different cells and growth factors play a role in the healing process. As our understanding of the process at cellular level improves, the hope is that we can use tissue engineering to enhance the process.

Tissue Engineering and Gene Therapy

Tissue engineering involves the application of scientific principles toward creating living tissue to replace, repair, or augment diseased tissue.[31] Gene therapy is the transfer of a certain gene into a cell so that the cell translates the gene into a specific protein. Scaffolds to support tissue growth are a necessary component of tissue engineering. By using a gene-therapy, tissue-engineered approach, one can select growth factors with documented roles in tendon healing to improve the healing process of RC repairs and deliver them locally at physiological concentrations.

In addition to the naturally derived scaffolds discussed above, synthetic polymers, such as poly-L-lactic acid (PLLA) and polyglycolic acid (PGA), can also be used as scaffolds. SIS and dermal ECMs are attractive due to their remodeling potential, which allows for replacement with host tissue. Downsides include the incomplete removal of animal DNA elements from their matrices and concerns about the biomechanical properties of the new tendon formed in their place. Synthetic polymers can be designed for use in specific tissues and can be mass produced.[32] Studies have shown that both PGA and PLLA can serve as carriers of cells and extracellular matrix and can be used to deliver specific growth factors to sites of tendon repair.[33,34] Augmentation of these scaffolds with the use of cell therapy, growth factors, or gene therapy may result in faster tendon healing and more biomechanically normal tendon formation.

Cell therapy aims to improve and accelerate tendon healing by enhancing cellular activity at the repair site. The process begins with procuring, purifying, and culturing particular cells. These are then seeded onto a carrier (scaffold) and implanted into the repair site. Many different cell types can be incorporated into the scaffold. Studies to date have focused on the use of mesenchymal stem cells (MSCs), tenocytes, and fibroblasts due to the roles they play in tendon healing. Uncommitted MSCs can replicate as undifferentiated cells, with the potential to differentiate toward tendon tissue.[35] Several studies have been done, assessing the effects of MSC implantation into tendon defects.[35,36] In one study, the material properties of MSC-based repairs were up to 33% better than control repairs.[37] Butler et al[36] showed that by 4 weeks, tendon repairs treated with MSCs exhibited twice the structural properties of contralateral controls and 50 to 60% of the stiffness and strength of normal tendons that were not surgically treated.

Growth factors are proteins that stimulate cell migration and proliferation as well as the synthesis of new tissue.[38] As outlined above, several growth factors are critical to the tendon repair process. Gene therapy can be used to induce local production of these growth factors. Gene therapy involves the transfer of a gene construct into a cell. The cell is then instructed to translate this into mRNA, thus overexpressing specific cytokines that play key roles in the healing process. Although the use of tissue engineering and gene therapy to enhance tendon healing holds promise; thus far, research has been limited to in vitro work and studies in small animal models. Further testing and long-term preclinical studies are needed until these applications can be deemed safe and beneficial for use in RC repairs in human beings.

The Future

Recently, our group presented data on the use of a novel, tissue engineering, gene therapy approach to RC tendon healing.[22] In part 1 of the study, we successfully transduced rat tendon fibroblasts with two different growth factors (IGF-1, PDGF-β) via retroviral vector. These transduced cells were then seeded onto a PGA scaffold, and their effect on nontransduced local responder cells was calculated. IGF-1-transduced cells stimulated collagen synthesis by 30% over controls and DNA synthesis by over 100% compared with controls. PDGF-β-transduced cells increased collagen synthesis more than 300% versus controls (**Fig. 14–2**). Based on these results, we evaluated the use of the gene-enhanced, tissue-engineered patch in a rat model of RC tendon tears.

RC tears were surgically created in adult Sprague Dawley rats. Two weeks later, the tears were repaired with suture alone (control) or with suture + PGA scaffold with IGF-1 or PDGF-β incorporated. Histologically, both experimental groups demonstrated qualitative improvements in repair, with better organization of tendon fiber bundles and evidence of neovascularization (**Fig. 14–3**). Biomechanically, our results demonstrated that IGF-1-enhanced repairs were significantly better ($p < 0.05$) in terms of max-

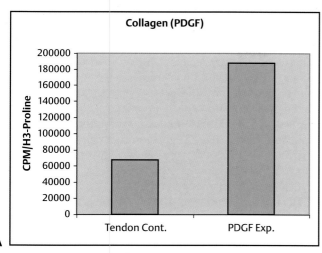

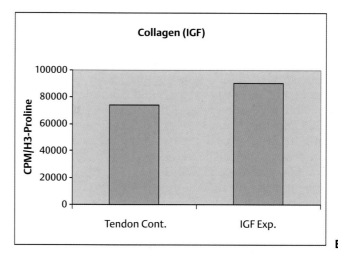

Figure 14–2 Increased collagen synthesis in experimental subjects versus controls. **(A)** Platelet-derived growth factor-β (PDGF-β). **(B)** Insulin-like growth factor-1 (IGF-1).

imum deformation and load to failure than controls and the PDGF-β-enhanced group. Results of this study indicate that IGF-1 enhanced RC tendon repairs in a small animal model. Clearly, further studies are necessary before this becomes a viable treatment option for human being RC tendon tears, but it does provide promise that we may be able to use biology to enhance surgery in the future.

Other Considerations: Muscle Degeneration

To date, most work regarding surgical improvement of RC repairs has focused on ensuring tendon healing to their insertions on the anatomic footprint of the greater tuberosity. Another consideration that must be addressed, if one is to maximize function after RC repairs, involves the possibility to reversing the well-documented, fatty muscle degen-

eration that occurs in the muscle bellies of the RC muscles after tendon tears.[39] Uthoff et al[40] used a rabbit model to see if early reattachment (6-weeks status postdetachment of the supraspinatus tendon) would reverse fat accumulation and muscle atrophy in the supraspinatus. They found that although fat accumulation and atrophy could not be reversed, earlier repair (compared with later reattachment) prevented an increase in fat accumulation. Gerber's group found similar results in a sheep model.[41] They showed that muscle atrophy and infiltration by fat cells led to impairment of the physiological properties of the muscle, which were irreversible in their experimental model.

Engineering skeletal muscle tissue that can generate controlled and efficient mechanical power would be extremely valuable toward achieving excellent results after RC repairs. However, there are few reports in the literature that address this issue.[42,43] In contrast to tendons, which contain ~70% extracellular matrix, skeletal muscle has a much

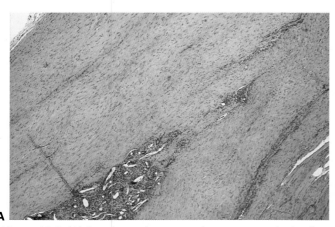

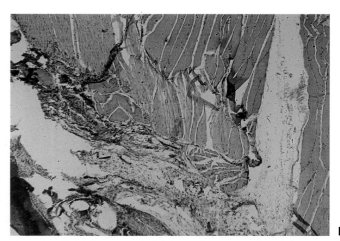

Figure 14–3 (A) Experimental group tendon; note organized collagen orientation (H&E, low power). **(B)** Control group tendon; disorganized collagen, increased vascularity.

smaller percentage of ECM (~5%).[44] Therefore, the ideal scaffold used to regenerate skeletal muscle would have at least 95% void space that could be occupied with cells. In addition, skeletal muscle is highly organized as a result of myocyte migration, alignment, and fusion; a process that most scaffolds do not allow.[41] Another obstacle to the use of scaffolds to regenerate skeletal muscle tissue stems from the fact that scaffolds function as a force shunt that "results in a derangement of the transmission of mechanical signals to individual muscle fibers ... which inhibits the generation of active contractile force . . . [and] interferes with the primary function of muscle as a tissue."[44] Other technological challenges exist including the establishment of adequate vascular supply to the muscle, the development of a functioning neuromuscular junction interface, and a functioning musculotendinous junction that facilitates force transmission. The successful engineering of skeletal muscle involves all of the above issues and is years away from being a viable clinical option. Nevertheless, the ability to regenerate such tissue would be extremely beneficial in terms of improving patients' outcomes after the repair of massive RC tears.

Summary

Despite improvements in our understanding and treatment of RC tears, our ability to get surgically repaired tendons to heal is still only satisfactory at best. Results for massive cuff tear repairs are even worse.[42] Thus far, FDA-approved ECMs[5] have been the only tool in the surgeon's armamentarium to potentially enhance repairs. Despite good results in small animal studies, the limited clinical studies in human beings have been less promising. Clearly, new therapies using tissue engineering and gene therapy are needed, which will help regenerate normal tendon tissue after repair. Again, promising results have been seen in small animal and in vitro models. However, many issues such as the ideal genes/cells to use, timing, and method of delivery, and the safety of such techniques must be addressed.

The ideal scaffold would be an off-the-shelf device that would provide some initial mechanical strength, be non-immunogenic, and highly conductive to cell infiltration. Furthermore, it would be bioabsorbable and not impede the normal repair process while degrading. The scaffold would contain a growth factor or morphogen capable of being a chemoattractant, as well as a stimulant for collagen synthesis. Although this may appear to be a futuristic goal, in reality, the foundations of such a strategy have already been laid.

Acknowledgment

The authors wish to thank Joseph Ianotti, M.D., Ph.D., for his generous contribution to this manuscript.

References

1. Gartsman GM, Khan M, Hammerman SM. Arthroscopic repair of full-thickness tears of the rotator cuff. J Bone Joint Surg Am 1998;80A(6):832–840
2. Rokito AS, Cuomo F, Gallagher MA, Zuckerman JD. Long-term functional outcome of repair of large and massive chronic tears of the rotator cuff. J Bone Joint Surg Am 1999;81A(7):991–997
3. Food and Drug Administration. Summary of safety and effectiveness, 2003. Available at: www.fda.gov/cdrh/pdf3/k0311969.pdf. Accessed .
4. Dejardin L, Arnoczky S, Ewers B, Haut R, Clarke R. Tissue-engineered rotator cuff tendon using procine small intestine submucosa: histologic and mechanical evaluation in dogs. Am J Sports Med 2001;29:175–184
5. Galatz LM, Ball CM, Teefey SA, Yamaguchi K. Outcome and repair integrity of completely arthroscopically repaired large and massive rotator cuff tears. J Bone Joint Surg Am 2004;86A(2):219–224
6. Postel JM, Goutallier D, Lavau L, Bernageau J. Anatomical results of rotator cuff repairs: study of 57 cases controlled by arthrography. J Shoulder Elbow Surg 1994;3:20
7. Derwin K, Baker A, Spragg K, Leigh D, Iannotti JP. Commercial extracellular matrix scaffolds for rotator cuff tendon repair: biomechanical, biochemical, and cellular properties. J Bone Joint Surg Am 2006; 88:2265–2272
8. Zheng M, Chen J, Kirilak Y, Willers C, Xu J, Wood D. Porcine small intestine submucosa is not an acellular collagenous matrix and contains porcine DNA: possible implications in human implantation. J Biomed Mater Res B Appl Biomat 2005;73(1):61–67
9. Hodde J, Badylak S, Brightman A, Voytik-Harbin S. Glycosaminoglycan content of small intestine submucosa: a bioscaffold for tissue replacement. Tissue Eng 1996;2(3):209–217
10. Rovak J, Bishop D, Boxer L, Wood S, Mungara A, Cederna P. Peripheral nerve transplantation: the role of chemical acellurization in eliminating allograft antigenicity. J Reconstr Microsurg 2005;21(3):207–213
11. Ketchedijan A, Jones A, Kreuger P, et al. Recellularization of decellularized allograft scaffolds in ovine great vessel reconstructions. Ann Thorac Surg 2005;79(3):888–896
12. Choe J, Bell T. Genetic Material is Present in Cadaveric Dermis and Cadaveric Fasica Lata. J Urol 2001;166(1):122–124
13. Iannotti J, Codsi M, Kwon Y, Derwin K, Ciccone J, Brems J. Porcine small intestine submucosa augmentation of surgical repair of chronic two tendon rotator cuff tears. J Bone Joint Surg Am 2006; 88:1238–1244
14. Malcarney H, Bonar F, Murrell G. Early inflammatory reaction after rotator cuff repair with a porcine small intestine submucosal implant: a report of 4 cases. Am J Sports Med 2005;33(6):907–911
15. Clarke K, Lantz G, Salisbury S, et al. Intestine submucosa and polypropylene mesh for abdominal wall repair in dogs. J Surg Res 1996;60:107–114
16. Sandusky G, Lantz G, Badylak S. Healing comparison of small intestine submucosa and eptfe grafts in the canine carotid artery. J Surg Res 1995;58:415–420
17. Kropp B, Badylak S, Thor K. Regenerative bladder augmentation: a review of initial preclinical studies with procine small intestine submucosa. Adv Exp Med Biol 1995;385:229–235

18. Zalavras C, Gardocki R, Huang E, et al. Reconstruction of large rotator cuff tendon defects with porcine small intestinal submucosa in an animal model. J Shoulder Elbow Surg 2006;15:224–231

19. Sclamberg SG, Tibone JE, Itamura JM, Kasraeian S. Six month MRI follow-up of large and massive rotator cuff repairs reinforced with porcine small intestinal submucosa. J Shoulder Elbow Surg 2004;13(5):538–541

20. Woo S, An K, Frank C. Anatomy, biology, and biomechanics of tendon and ligament. In: Burkwalter JA, Einhorn TA, Simon SR, eds. Orthopaedic Basic Science. 2nd ed. Rosemont IL; 2000:582–614

21. Kobayashi K, Hamada K, Gotoh M, Handa A, Yamakawa H, Fukuda H. Healing of full-thickness tears of avian supracoracoid tendons: in situ hybridization of a1(I) and a1(III) procollagen mRNA. J Orthop Res 2001;19:862–868

22. Dines JS, Grande D, Dines DM. Tissue engineering and rotator cuff tendon healing. J Shoulder Elbow Surg 2007;16(55):S204–S207

23. Lewis C, Schlegel T, Hawkins R, Turner S. The effects of immobilization on rotator cuff healing using modified mason allen stitches: a biomechanical study in sheep. Biomed Sci Instrum 2001;37:263–268

24. Bey M, Ramsey M, Soslowsky L. Intratendinous train field of the supraspinatus tendon: effect of a surgically created articular-surface rotator cuff tear. J Shoulder Elbow Surg 2002;11(6):562–569

25. Thomopoulos S, Hattersley G, Rose V, et al. The localized expression of extracellular matrix components in healing tendon insertion sites: an in situ hybridization study. J Orthop Res 2002;20:454–463

26. Skutek M, van Griensven M, Zeichen J, Brauer N, Bosch U. Cyclic mechanical stretching modulates secretion pattern of growth factors in human tendon fibroblasts. Eur J Appl Physiol 2001;86(1):48–52

27. Aspenburg P, Forslund C. Enhanced tendon healing with GDF-5 and 6. Acta Orthop Scand 1999;70(1):51–54

28. Nakase T, Sugamoto K, Miyamoto T, et al. Activation of cartilage derived morphogenic protein-1 in torn rotator cuff. Clin Orthop Relat Res 2002;399:140–145

29. Yoshikawa Y, Abrahamsson SO. Dose-related cellular effects of platelet–derived growth factor-BB differ in various types of rabbit tendons in vitro. Acta Orthop Scand 2001;72(3):287–292

30. Dahlgren LA, van der Meulen MC, Bertram JE, Starrak GS, Nixon AJ. Insulin-like growth factor-I improves cellular and molecular aspects of healing in a collagenase-induced model of flexor tendinitis. J Orthop Res 2002;20(5):910–919

31. Huard J, Fu F, eds. Gene Therapy and Tissue Engineering in Orthopaedic and Sports Medicine. Boston: Birkhauser; 2000

32. Musgrave D, Fu F, Huard J. Gene therapy and tissue engineering in orthopaedic surgery. J Am Acad Orthop Surg 2002;10(1):6–15

33. Athanasiou K, Niederauer C, Agrawal C. Sterilization, toxicity, biocompatability and clinical applications of polylactic acid/polyglycolic acid copolymers. Biomaterials 1996;17:93–102

34. Pittenger M, Mackay A, Beck S, et al. Multilineage potential of adult human mesenchymal stem cells. Science 1999;284:143–147

35. Butler D, Awad H. Perspectives on cell and collagen composites for tendon repair. Clin Orthop Relat Res 1999;367S:S324–S332

36. Awad H, Butler D, Boivin G, et al. Autologous mesenchymal stem cell-mediated tendon repair. Tissue Eng 1999;5:267–277

37. Lindberg K, Badylak S. A bioscaffold supporting in vitro primary human epidermal cell differentiation and synthesis of basement membrane proteins. Burns 2001;27:254–266

38. Goutallier D, Postel J, Bernageau J, Lavau L, Voisin M. Fatty muscle degeneration in cuff ruptures. Pre and postoperative evaluation by CT scan. Clin Orthop Relat Res 1994;304:78–83

39. Uthoff H, Matsumoto F, Trudel G, Himori K. Early reattachment does not reverse atrophy and fat accumulation of the suprapinatus-an experimental study in rabbits. J Orthop Res 2003;21(3):386–392

40. Gerber C, Meyer D, Schneeberger A, Hoppeler H, von Rechenberg B. Effect of tendon release and delayed repair on the structure of the muscles of the rotator cuff: an experimental study in sheep. J Bone Joint Surg Am 2004;86A(9):1973–1982

41. Dennis R, Kosnik PE. Excitability and isometric contractile properties of mammalian skeletal muscle constructs engineered in vitro. In Vitro Cell Dev Biol Anim 2000;36:327–335

42. Dennis R, Kosnik PE, Gilbert ME, Faulkner JA. Excitability and contractility of skeletal muscle engineered from primary cultures and cell lines. Am J Physiol Cell Physiol 2001;280:C288–C295

43. Dennis R. Tissue engineering in muscle: current challenges and directions. In: Sandell L, Grodzinsky A, eds. Tissue Engineering in Musculoskeletal Clinical Practice. Rosemont, IL: American Academy of Orthopedic Surgeons; 2003:95–301

44. Hodde J, Record R, Liang H, Badylak S. Vascular endothelial growth factor in porcine derived extracellular matrix. Endothelium 2001;8(1):11–24

Index

Page numbers followed by *f* or *t* indicate material in figures or tables respectively.